P9-DGH-780

the Beck DIET solution
Weight Loss Workbook

Judith S. Beck, Ph.D.

Beck Institute for Cognitive Therapy and Research

Clinical Associate Professor of Psychology in Psychiatry

University of Pennsylvania

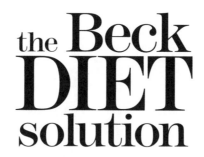

the **Beck
DIET**
solution

Weight Loss Workbook

The 6-Week Plan to Train Your Brain to Think Like a Thin Person

- *counteract sabotaging thoughts*
- *overcome weight loss obstacles*
- *succeed on any nutritious diet*

Judith S. Beck, Ph.D.

Beck Institute for Cognitive Therapy and Research
Clinical Associate Professor of Psychology in Psychiatry
University of Pennsylvania

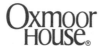

Oxmoor
House®

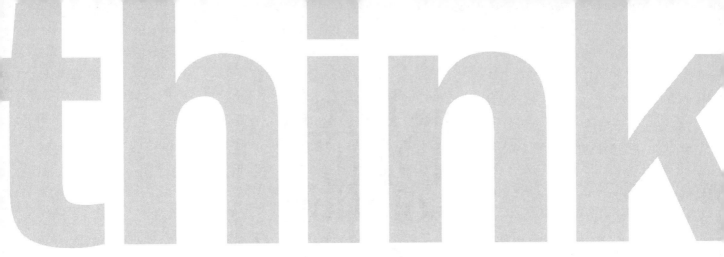

©2007 by Judith S. Beck, Ph.D.

All rights reserved. No part of this book may be reproduced in any form or by any means without the prior written permission of the publisher, excepting brief quotations in connection with reviews written specifically for inclusion in magazines or newspapers, or limited excerpts strictly for personal use.

Published by Oxmoor House, an imprint of Time Inc. Books
225 Liberty Street, New York, NY 10281

ISBN-13: 978-0-8487-3191-5
ISBN-10: 0-8487-3191-3
Printed in the United States of America
Seventh Printing 2017

Be sure to check with your health-care provider before making any changes in your diet.

Editorial and Production Support: Allison Long Lowery, L. Amanda Owens, Melissa Jones Clark, Amelia Heying, Rachel Quinlivan, Laura Lockhart, Greg A. Amason, Faye Porter Bonner

To order additional publications, call 1-800-765-6400.

To my family and Naomi

Contents

How the Beck Diet Solution Works

The Program

chapter 5

Week 1: Create a Foundation for Diet Success   38

chapter 6
Week 2: **Get Ready for Dieting**   52

chapter 7
Week 3: **Let the Diet Begin!**   84

chapter 8
Week 4: **Fight Undermining Ideas**   122

chapter 9

Week 5: **Solve Real-life Problems**   164

chapter 10

Week 6: **Hone Your New Skills**   205

Transition from Losing to Maintaining

Acknowledgments

So many people to thank!

First, thanks to my husband, Richard Busis, for his unending support, enthusiasm, and encouragement. To Naomi Dank, my wonderful friend and colleague, for her generosity of time, effort, and spirit, and to Phyllis Beck, my wonderful mother, for her unflagging nurturance and sage advice. To Aaron Beck, my gifted father, who pioneered the field of Cognitive Therapy and taught me so much. To Deborah Beck Busis, my daughter, who has helped me develop and refine this Cognitive Therapy approach to weight-loss management. To my other children, Samuel Beck Busis and Sarah Beck Busis, and Sarah's husband, Matthew Cohen, who always enrich my life.

Thanks to those consummate professionals whose help has been instrumental in so many ways: Brian Carnahan, Amanda Owens, Linda Barker, Melissa Clark, and Karen Kelly.

Thanks also to two exceptionally talented women who have nourished my work and me: my agent, Stephanie Tade, and my publicist, Beth Grossman.

Finally, I would like to extend my gratitude to those who provided us with feedback about the original book, *The Beck Diet Solution:* dieters with whom Debbie Busis and I have worked directly and the hundreds and hundreds of people who have e-mailed us or posted on Internet blogs, bulletin boards, and discussion groups. Your input continues to inspire and influence our work.

think

How the Beck Diet Solution Works

Introduction to the Beck Diet Solution

T he Beck Diet Solution is a six-week program that teaches you a different psychological skill every day to help you achieve your weight-loss goals. Both the original book, *The Beck Diet Solution,* and this workbook are different from any other diet-related books you've ever read. For starters, they don't include a diet plan! Also, they don't tell you *what* to eat or even *when* to eat. Instead, the Beck Diet Solution program teaches you all of the skills you need to be able to stick to any nutritious diet of your choice, to lose excess weight, and to keep it off for your lifetime.

These skills are based on the principles of Cognitive Therapy, which is one of the most common—and powerful—psychotherapies practiced worldwide today. Demonstrated in hundreds of research studies to be effective in the treatment of a variety of psychological problems, Cognitive Therapy focuses on helping you change your thinking so that you can maintain lifelong changes in your behavior.

Why haven't you been successful with dieting in the past? If you're like most people, you think that the only preparation you need to do is to pick a diet plan—and you're ready to get started. And, actually, dieting can be pretty easy at first. You're highly motivated, and you can temporarily make changes in your eating habits to lose weight without much trouble. A week or two goes by, and you feel successful and in control. You're losing weight. You're happy.

But you've been fooled.

Because the first few days or weeks of your diet are relatively easy, you naturally think that eating less, resisting cravings, and handling hunger will *always* be easy. Wrong! Sooner or later, it's going to become more difficult for you to stick to your plan and to say no to some of your favorite foods. You'll have a "sabotaging thought," such as, *It's okay if I eat this food [that I'm not supposed to eat] because....* (You can fill in the blank with dozens of excuses.) Then what happens? You give in, and before you know it, you've gained back the excess weight you lost. But it doesn't have to be that way! This workbook teaches you exactly what to say to yourself and exactly what to do to get back on track *immediately.*

Key Components of the Beck Diet Solution

Talking back to sabotaging thoughts is essential to weight-loss success. You will most likely have lots of these thoughts on the way to achieving your goal. For example, figure out what you're thinking as you read this list of important features of the Beck Diet Solution program:

- Pick a nutritious diet and a reasonable exercise program.
- Plan and monitor in writing what you eat.
- Use good eating habits so that you really notice and enjoy every bite.
- Solve diet- and exercise-related problems.
- Transition to rest-of-your-life eating and exercising.

Do you have such thoughts as, *I don't want to do that,* or, *I don't have to do that*? It's exactly these kinds of thoughts that you will learn how to effectively respond to so that you'll be motivated to do what's needed to lose weight and to keep it off.

I'll bet that no one ever taught you *how* to do all these things. It's not surprising that dieting has been difficult for you. You didn't have all these essential skills!

Learning to Diet Is Like Learning to Play Tennis

If you're still not convinced that you need skills to lose weight and not just a diet plan, the following analogy may help: Let's say you've decided to take up tennis. You can't expect to just pick up a racket and win a game. You need a coach, someone to teach you exactly what to do. Having the right mindset is also important. You have to recognize that it takes time, energy, and effort to perfect your tennis skills. You have to practice them over and over—and, in time, tennis will get easier and easier. But you still can't expect to win every game. Even if you're a good player, there will be days when you make mistakes. Realizing this ahead of time makes it easier to handle your disappointment when you lose a game.

Imagine if you had unrealistic expectations: if you truly believed that you *should* be able to figure out how to play on your own, if you thought instruction and practice were unimportant, if you expected yourself to play exceptionally well every day—and that there's something wrong with you if you had difficulty. You'd get upset and think, *I thought I could play tennis ... I guess I was wrong ... I can't.* At that point, you might abandon playing tennis altogether.

The same principles hold for dieting. You can probably choose a diet plan, start following it right away, and lose some weight. But, at some point, it's going to get more difficult—and if you don't know what to do, you're likely to get demoralized, give up, and start gaining back weight. This workbook prepares you for those difficult times. It teaches you exactly what to say to yourself and what to do so that *this time* you will keep losing excess weight and keep down your weight for life.

If you've read *The Beck Diet Solution,* think of this introduction and chapters 1–4 of this workbook as an intensive refresher course in the program. Don't skim over these sections. There's plenty of new material and a weight-loss questionnaire that sheds light on why you have dieting difficulties. If you haven't read the original book, I want you to know that it's helpful to do so but not essential. You'll still benefit from the ideas, techniques, and daily charts in this interactive companion. As you make your way through this workbook, you're going to learn exciting new weight-loss strategies. No wonder you haven't been able to lose weight or to keep it off—you didn't know *how*. But now you have the opportunity to learn, and I'm very glad you decided to join me in this journey.

chapter 1

How Cognitive Therapy Helps You Achieve Lasting Weight Loss

The Beck Diet Solution is grounded in the principles of Cognitive Therapy (CT). *Cognitive* refers to thinking. In the late 1950s and early 1960s, my father, Aaron T. Beck, M.D., developed this form of "talk therapy" as a result of a number of scientific experiments he conducted. He found that when he helped depressed patients solve their current problems and modify their unrealistic and depressed thoughts, they started to feel better and behave in more helpful ways. Instead of spending *years* talking about their childhood experiences "on the couch," he had patients sit up, set goals for treatment, and learn skills to change their behavior *and* thinking. Patients got better quickly, often in just 10 to 12 sessions.

Over 400 research studies have shown CT to be effective for a wide range of problems and disorders. A recent study conducted in Sweden demonstrated the effectiveness of CT for weight loss. Researchers reported on the outcome of dieters who participated in a 10-week group CT treatment program and returned for a follow-up 18 months after treatment ended. These dieters initially lost an average of 18 pounds. A year and a half later, on average they had continued to lose several more pounds each. (A different group who did not receive CT actually gained weight during this same period.) These results are truly impressive.

Why was the CT program so successful? After all, statistics show that even if they lose weight most people regain it within a year. One key ingredient in all CT treatments is an emphasis on helping people change their thinking so that they can change their actions. A key feature of this workbook is its emphasis on teaching you how to identify and respond forcefully to unhelpful thoughts that sabotage your dieting efforts. You'll learn the tools you need to do everything that is necessary to lose excess weight and to keep it off permanently.

How Your Thinking Can Lead You Astray

Think back to the last time you deviated from a diet, when you ate something you knew you weren't supposed to. Was it some kind of junk food that your diet plan did not allow? Or did you eat some permitted food in a much greater quantity than allowed? What did you say to give yourself permission to eat it? It's amazing how creative our minds can be when we really want to do something we shouldn't. Chances are, you thought something such as, *It's okay to eat this because … I'm stressed/I'm hungry/I just don't care/I really want it/everyone else is having it/it looks so good/I can't resist it/it won't matter/I'll start my diet again tomorrow/it's free/no one is watching/I'm celebrating.*

You probably realize how faulty this kind of thinking is now. You recognize that it's not okay to eat at these times if you want to lose weight. But sabotaging thoughts can be quite compelling while you're having them. Fortunately, there are powerful tools to counteract these unhelpful thoughts.

Why Eating Can Seem Automatic—But Isn't

Do you believe that sometimes your eating is involuntary, that you're not thinking anything when you put food in your mouth? For instance, when you were stressed, did you ever eat a whole pint of ice cream without even noticing? That kind of eating may *seem* automatic and involuntary, but it isn't. Biological functions—such as the beating of your heart and the digestion of food—are automatic. But eating is *not*. You *always* make a decision to eat or not to eat, to keep eating or to stop eating.

Here's another way of looking at this: Let's say that you're watching a DVD at a friend's house. On the coffee table in front of you is a plate of large cookies, some napkins, and a few round coasters. You planned to eat just one cookie while you watched the movie.

But before you know it, you've eaten three of them. You didn't eat them automatically. *You thought about it first.* After all, if eating were automatic and required no thought, why didn't you pick up the coasters that were the same size and eat them? No, you thought about picking up each cookie, even if you weren't fully aware of your thoughts at the time.

The reason that eating sometimes *seems* automatic is that you're paying more attention to other things. Sometimes, this lack of focus is unintentional; you're distracted by conversation or by other environmental stimuli. At other times, you may intentionally try not to notice how much you're eating. But you're not completely distracted in either case. At some level, you know that you're continuing to put food in your mouth. Thank goodness! If eating really were automatic, you wouldn't be able to do anything about it.

Triggers and the Eating Process

The thoughts you have about eating don't come out of nowhere. There's always a trigger that precedes your thoughts. For example, you see a bag of pretzels when you open your cabinet to get out something else. Seeing the pretzels is the trigger. You then have some thoughts, such as, *These look good ... I think I'll have some.* Then you reach up, get the bag, open it, and put the pretzels in your mouth. Triggers do not automatically lead to eating, though. Your *thoughts* determine whether or not you actually eat.

Below are five categories of triggers. Check off the ones that you've experienced:

☐ **Biological:** hunger pangs, thirst, hormonally influenced cravings, or other biological processes

☐ **Environmental:** seeing or smelling food, watching a cooking program or food commercial

☐ **Mental:** thinking about food (for example, realizing it is almost lunchtime), imagining eating some wonderful food, having a positive memory of some wonderful food you ate in the past, or a negative memory of being hungry or deprived

☐ **Emotional:** tension, anxiety, sadness, loneliness, boredom, and other negative emotions; also positive emotions, such as happiness or excitement

☐ **Social:** being offered food or being around people who are eating

Some triggers are obvious: You pass a pizza shop and smell the wonderful aroma emanating from it. Some are not: You crave chocolate and don't realize that you've been stimulated by hormones. Fortunately, it's not critical to be able to identify the trigger that leads you to eat. It is helpful, however, to be able to predict what's likely to trigger you so that you can minimize your exposure, especially at the beginning of your diet. But no matter what the trigger is, you're going to follow the same sequence to resist giving in to food you're not supposed to eat.

Dieters' Thinking Versus Thin Thinking

What makes it difficult to resist any kind of trigger is your sabotaging thinking. There are some very interesting differences in how unsuccessful dieters think compared with those who have successfully maintained their weight loss through the Beck Diet Solution program. Both experience the same kinds of triggers. But unsuccessful dieters have certain characteristics and ways of thinking that can lead to failure, as illustrated in the chart on the facing page.

Identifying Thoughts

At this point, you may not be aware of your thoughts just before you eat. In fact, often they last just a millisecond. You may simply think something such as, *I want to eat that.* Later in the program, you'll learn how to identify your thoughts. But you can start practicing this skill right now, if you'd like. Whenever you have the desire to eat, ask yourself, *What's going through my mind right now? What am I thinking?*

Don't worry if you have difficulty doing this at first. I'll present numerous examples of sabotaging thoughts throughout the workbook, and the skill of combating them will get easier and easier for you.

Thinking Differences Chart

Characteristics of Unsuccessful Dieters	Thinking of Unsuccessful Dieters	Thinking of Successful Maintainers
Confusion between hunger and desire to eat	*I just ate dinner half an hour ago, but I'm starving! I have to have a snack.*	*I'm not hungry; I'm just having a craving. I don't need those cookies.*
Intolerance of hunger	*I can't stand being hungry.*	*Hunger is mildly uncomfortable, but I can tolerate it. It will go away if I focus on something else.*
Desire for overfullness	*If I eat a lot, I'll be more satisfied and won't run the risk of getting hungry.*	*It's okay if I get hungry. I'd rather get a little hungry and stay thinner than eat a lot and gain weight.*
Self-deception	*It doesn't really matter if I eat this extra food.*	*It does matter. If I eat it, I'll strengthen the habit of giving in, which will make it more likely that I'll give in again next time ... and the next ... and the next.*
Eating as an emotional coping strategy	*I'm upset. If I eat, I'll feel better. I deserve to indulge myself.*	*If I eat, I'll have two problems: the one that was upsetting in the first place and now feeling bad about myself. I'm going to be very sorry in a few minutes if I eat now.*
Demoralization upon weight gain	*I can't believe I gained weight! This is terrible! I just can't lose weight. Maybe I should just give up.*	*Oh, well, I gained a little weight. I'll just be more careful this week.*
Focus on unfairness	*It's so unfair that other people can eat what they want and I can't.*	*I'm so glad I'm not eating like everyone else. I'd much rather be thinner.*

chapter 2

Get Ready to Begin the Program

Before you even get started on the Beck Diet Solution program, I would like you to first do the following things: select a diet coach, pick a healthy eating plan (in fact, you'll pick two—I'll tell you why on page 24!), and choose a sound exercise program. Start with finding a supportive coach so that he/she can consult with you in deciding on a nutritious diet and a doable exercise program.

Choosing a Diet Coach

Some dieters are reluctant to approach someone—often a trusted friend or close family member—about being a diet coach. I hope you won't feel embarrassed, as some dieters are, to ask someone to be your coach. It's truly wonderful that you're making the effort to lose excess weight; it's admirable, not shameful. I also hope you're not concerned about imposing on someone. Many people actually feel honored when they're asked to help. Being a diet coach isn't very time consuming. You'll arrange to call (or see) your coach once a week to report your progress and to e-mail or call in between whenever you need extra help.

Whom should you pick to be your diet coach? He/she doesn't need to be experienced in dieting, just someone who is supportive and a good problem-solver. Here are a few suggestions:

- A friend, family member, coworker, or member of your community

- A fellow dieter from an organized diet support group

- A diet professional

- An Internet support diet buddy

I'd like you to line up a diet coach now, even though you probably would be okay without one for the first few days or weeks of the program. In my experience, dieters are less likely to look for help when they start having problems, so it's best to have someone to whom you've been talking regularly. You're going to ask your coach to help you stay motivated, build your confidence, and solve problems. You're going to keep yourself accountable by reporting your change in weight (not necessarily your actual weight) to your coach every week.

Choosing Your Diet

While I don't recommend any particular diet plan over another, I do strongly urge you to select one that is *healthy* and *reasonable,* which allows you to eat a variety of whole, fresh foods (fruits, vegetables, grains, lean protein, some unsaturated fat), gives you enough nutrients, and is not too calorie restrictive (many health professionals recommend that you eat from 1,200 to 1,600 calories a day). It's also important to choose a plan with meals that you can easily prepare and that you like.

There are two basic kinds of diets: One provides a set plan (telling you specifically what and how much to eat, as well as providing menus for you to follow); the other requires you to calculate the foods you eat according to a system (calories, carbs, assigned points, or units). Some are a combination of the two. The diet you choose should be relatively simple to follow (complicated meal planning or diets that require you to make special foods or follow elaborate recipes are often too frustrating to maintain over time) and, most importantly, healthy (grapefruit diets and cabbage soup regimens might work for a few days, but they certainly aren't healthy or sustainable over the long term).

before you begin:

Check with a Medical Professional

Everyone needs to check with his/her health-care professional as soon as a diet plan has been selected—but before starting it—to make sure the diet is safe and nutritionally sound. You also need to confirm that your exercise plan will be safe and effective for you.

Pros and Cons of Diet Methods

All diet plans have positive and negative aspects. It's worth reviewing what these aspects are before you decide on your diet plan.

Diet Methods Chart	
Set Plans	**Counting Plans**
Advantages:	**Advantages:**
You are provided with menus—and often recipes—for each meal. You don't have to make lots of food decisions, and you don't have to count calories or units of food. You know what has to go on your shopping list and how to prepare your food. It's very clear what and how much you should eat at each meal.	You create your own menus and have more choices so you can prepare the kinds of foods you enjoy. It may be easier to eat out. You can buy foods in season and on sale, so these diets work well if you're on a budget or want to do your best to eat foods that are fresh, seasonal, and local.
Disadvantages:	**Disadvantages:**
You have fewer food choices. You have to eat as directed. If you don't have control over your food intake (for example, because you're traveling or eating out), you sometimes may have to deviate from the plan. You may be directed to eat some foods that you don't particularly enjoy.	You have to be careful to make sure you eat nutritiously. You could use your calories on unhealthy food, which can set you up for intense hunger and cravings. In addition to counting calories, you'll need to spend more time planning meals and selecting the right foods for nutritional balance.

Keeping Track of Calories and Portion Sizes

It's important for you to be aware of your intake of calories, even if your diet plan doesn't require you to count them. To lose weight, you have to eat fewer calories than you burn. If your diet plan allows you to eat an unlimited amount of certain foods, you can become accustomed to large portion sizes and end up ingesting too many calories.

Modifying Your Diet Plan

Now, let's talk about whether you can realistically follow the diet plan you choose over the long run. If your diet forbids you to eat certain foods, is it realistic for you to expect that you'll never have them again? I don't want you to set yourself up for failure. I want you to start thinking now of what modifications you should make to your diet plan so you can follow it long term.

For example, you might want to eat a little bit of junk food every day, as I do. If junk food isn't on your plan, you can still decide to have a small portion, as long as you figure out how many calories it has and reduce your intake of other food accordingly. Just be careful that you're not unduly skimping on healthy food, or your body will rebel, making it very difficult to sustain your diet. And figure out precisely when you're going to eat this restricted food. You may decide, as I have, to eat it only as an evening snack—and not at any other times. I don't want you to decide on the spur of the moment whether or not to modify your diet. That's a recipe for disaster. Make a reasonable decision now, before you start. Ask your diet coach to help you figure this out.

Another diet modification you might want to make is in the number of times you eat per day. Regardless of what your diet plan recommends, what is best for you? Some people do better to eat just three meals a day, with no snacks. Others do better to have three smaller meals a day in addition to one, two, or three snacks. Whatever you decide, make sure to have breakfast, lunch, and dinner at a minimum. Don't skip meals!

What About Prepackaged Foods?

One kind of set plan involves eating prepackaged meals that you can obtain from a commercial weight-loss program or buy at the supermarket. Doing so can help you learn about appropriate portion sizes. And these meals certainly make life easier. So it's fine to begin in this way (unless you have a medical condition that necessitates a reduction of salt or additives).

The downside to eating prepackaged foods is that it may not fit into your lifestyle (if you eat some meals out of the house); it limits your consumption of fresh foods that don't contain additives; and it just postpones the necessity to learn how to eat "normally," since it's not healthy (or economical) to eat prepackaged foods for the rest of your life.

Can I Still Eat Fast Food?

Ultimately, I want you to be flexible enough that you can plan to eat whatever foods you want, even fast food. You need to eat some foods in small quantities—and not too frequently—especially if they're high in calories and not very nutritious or if they contain ingredients that aren't good for your health. Toward the beginning of your diet, though, you can eat fast food *if* it's allowed by your food plan. Try it, if you want. Watch out for cravings, though. Many people are undone by the smell of French fries, for example, and eat them even if they're an unplanned item. I don't want to put too much temptation in your path initially. It's not that cravings are bad—but they *are* uncomfortable, so I'd like you to do what you can to minimize them.

Evaluating Your Diet Plan

Now that you've read about the different kinds of diet plans, it's time to investigate your options:

- Go to the bookstore or library.

- Call your health-care professional.

- Consult with other dieters who have been successful.

- Investigate commercial weight-loss programs.

- Check with your local hospital, gym, or community center for programs.

- Find a nutritionist.

- Go online.

When assessing various diets, you need to review them thoroughly and carefully. When you've selected a potential plan, complete this checklist:

yes no

☐ ☐ Are the requirements of this diet (for example, preparing specific meals or counting calories) easy for me to learn and to practice every day?

☐ ☐ Is this diet nutritious?

☐ ☐ Does it contain at least 1,200 to 1,600 calories a day?

☐ ☐ Does it allow me to easily choose foods that I like?

☐ ☐ Can I live with this plan—or a modification of the plan—for the long term?

If you answered yes to all of these questions, it's a diet worth pursuing. If you answered no to even one of the questions, there's a good chance you will find the diet difficult after a while.

After you select a diet, believe it or not I'd like you to choose *another* one. A number of dieters I've worked with became bored with their primary diet and, without a backup plan, would have simply stopped dieting entirely. I'd like you to decide now which diet you're going to switch to if this happens to you.

Choosing Your Exercise Program

Exercise burns calories, gives you energy, and improves your overall health. It's an important part of losing weight and maintaining weight loss—and an essential part of being as healthy as you can be. In the past, you might have considered exercise to be optional. Now, I'd like you to view it as mandatory.

One key to successfully adding exercise to your schedule is to choose something you like to do. It could be walking; hiking; running; working out at a gym; taking exercise, dance, or martial-arts classes; playing a sport; exercising to a DVD or TV program; swimming; or biking.

If you're not currently exercising, you will have to organize your life around exercise, instead of just "fitting it in" when you can. The only way exercise consistently happens is if you schedule it. You also may need backup plans if you've planned to exercise outside and the weather is bad.

Finally, in addition to your planned program, I'd like you to start looking for opportunities to fit "spontaneous exercise" into your day whenever you can. Here are some suggestions:

- Routinely take the stairs instead of the elevator.

- Park a distance away from your destination.

- Get off the bus several stops early.

- Pace the corridors of your building several times a day.

- Take your dog for extra walks.

- Turn on music and dance.

- Do a circuit of the entire mall or superstore before you begin shopping.

Now that you've learned some of the basics about selecting a diet coach, choosing healthy diets, and making exercise a priority, you're ready to learn more about yourself and your eating habits.

chapter 3

The Beck Diet Solution Questionnaire

Before you begin your diet plan, I'd like you to fill out this questionnaire, a modified version of which we give to the dieters we counsel at the Beck Institute for Cognitive Therapy. You'll answer the questionnaire again six weeks from now in a different color ink. I think you'll be surprised at how different your responses are after following this program.

This questionnaire is designed to make you think about your dieting history, motivation level, eating habits, reactions toward dieting, response to hunger and cravings, and reasons for overeating. Do your best when answering each question. Highlight any questions you're unsure of so that you can come back and answer them as you become more aware of your thoughts and behaviors in the coming weeks. For example, many people initially have difficulty answering the following question: How often do you try to avoid feeling hunger or cravings?

Diet History

- How many times have you tried to lose weight? _____

- How many times have you lost weight but gained some or all of it back? _____

- How satisfied are you with your current weight?
  ☐ Not at all   ☐ A little   ☐ A moderate amount   ☐ A lot   ☐ Completely

The reason I ask these questions is to impress the following idea on you: Whatever you've tried in the past didn't help enough or you would have lost weight and kept it off. If you're tempted to skip some tasks in this workbook, remind yourself that not learning, practicing, and using these techniques in the past hasn't gotten you where you want to be.

Motivation Level

- How willing are you to change your eating and exercise habits?
  ☐ Not at all   ☐ A little   ☐ A moderate amount   ☐ A lot   ☐ Completely

- How willing are you to tell relevant people you're changing the way you eat?
  ☐ Not at all   ☐ A little   ☐ A moderate amount   ☐ A lot   ☐ Completely

- How willing are you to put in the time needed to exercise, shop for foods listed on your diet plan, and prepare healthy foods?
  ☐ Not at all   ☐ A little   ☐ A moderate amount   ☐ A lot   ☐ Completely

If you're not completely willing to do these things, you will need to learn how to increase your motivation because these tasks are essential. Is there some reason you believe you can not only lose weight but also maintain your weight loss for your lifetime without doing these things?

Eating Habits

- How often do you eat standing up?
  ☐ Never   ☐ Rarely   ☐ Sometimes   ☐ Often   ☐ Always

- How often do you eat quickly?
  ☐ Never   ☐ Rarely   ☐ Sometimes   ☐ Often   ☐ Always

- How often do you forget to notice every bite you're eating?
  ☐ Never   ☐ Rarely   ☐ Sometimes   ☐ Often   ☐ Always

Don't worry if your answers to these questions make you realize that your eating habits need improvement. You'll learn how to get yourself to eat sitting down, as well as to slow down and notice every bite consistently.

Reactions Toward Dieting

- How often do you feel a sense of unfairness that you're not supposed to eat what or as much as others are eating?
  ☐ Never ☐ Rarely ☐ Sometimes ☐ Often ☐ Always

- How often do you get discouraged when you're dieting?
  ☐ Never ☐ Rarely ☐ Sometimes ☐ Often ☐ Always

- How often do you feel deprived?
  ☐ Never ☐ Rarely ☐ Sometimes ☐ Often ☐ Always

- How often do you feel that dieting is just too hard?
  ☐ Never ☐ Rarely ☐ Sometimes ☐ Often ☐ Always

- How often do you feel like dieting just isn't worth it?
  ☐ Never ☐ Rarely ☐ Sometimes ☐ Often ☐ Always

Most people who have failed at dieting have negative attitudes. You'll learn how to develop more helpful attitudes throughout this workbook.

Hunger and Cravings

- How often do you try to avoid feeling hunger or cravings (by eating past the point of just mild fullness or by eating snacks you hadn't planned on consuming)?
  ☐ Never ☐ Rarely ☐ Sometimes ☐ Often ☐ Always

- How often do you think, *I really* need *to eat something now?*
  ☐ Never ☐ Rarely ☐ Sometimes ☐ Often ☐ Always

- How often are you unsure if you're really hungry or not?
  ☐ Never ☐ Rarely ☐ Sometimes ☐ Often ☐ Always

Most dieters mix up hunger and cravings. They also believe that it's somehow bad to experience these sensations. You'll do experiments to demonstrate to yourself that hunger and cravings aren't bad, they're merely uncomfortable, they come and go, and you *can* learn to tolerate them.

Overeating

How often do you eat _more_ than you should when ...

- You're feeling down, nervous, lonely, frustrated, or annoyed.
  ☐ Never   ☐ Rarely   ☐ Sometimes   ☐ Often   ☐ Always

- You're bored.
  ☐ Never   ☐ Rarely   ☐ Sometimes   ☐ Often   ☐ Always

- You're trying to avoid or postpone doing something you know you should do.
  ☐ Never   ☐ Rarely   ☐ Sometimes   ☐ Often   ☐ Always

- You're tired.
  ☐ Never   ☐ Rarely   ☐ Sometimes   ☐ Often   ☐ Always

- You're not feeling well physically.
  ☐ Never   ☐ Rarely   ☐ Sometimes   ☐ Often   ☐ Always

- You're very hungry or experiencing cravings.
  ☐ Never   ☐ Rarely   ☐ Sometimes   ☐ Often   ☐ Always

Many people who struggle with losing weight eat in response to emotional or physical triggers. You'll learn in this workbook how to plan in advance what to do when you encounter these triggers.

When you see food you know you really shouldn't eat, how often do you think, _It's okay to eat this food because_ ...

- It's not a whole piece.
  ☐ Never   ☐ Rarely   ☐ Sometimes   ☐ Often   ☐ Always

- It's not that fattening.
  ☐ Never   ☐ Rarely   ☐ Sometimes   ☐ Often   ☐ Always

- I'll make up for it later.
  ☐ Never   ☐ Rarely   ☐ Sometimes   ☐ Often   ☐ Always

- I can start again tomorrow.
  ☐ Never   ☐ Rarely   ☐ Sometimes   ☐ Often   ☐ Always

- It won't matter this one time.
  ☐ Never   ☐ Rarely   ☐ Sometimes   ☐ Often   ☐ Always

- It will go to waste.
  ☐ Never   ☐ Rarely   ☐ Sometimes   ☐ Often   ☐ Always

- No one is watching.
  ☐ Never   ☐ Rarely   ☐ Sometimes   ☐ Often   ☐ Always

- I already paid for it.
  ☐ Never ☐ Rarely ☐ Sometimes ☐ Often ☐ Always

- I don't care.
  ☐ Never ☐ Rarely ☐ Sometimes ☐ Often ☐ Always

- I really want it.
  ☐ Never ☐ Rarely ☐ Sometimes ☐ Often ☐ Always

- I deserve a treat.
  ☐ Never ☐ Rarely ☐ Sometimes ☐ Often ☐ Always

- I'm celebrating.
  ☐ Never ☐ Rarely ☐ Sometimes ☐ Often ☐ Always

- I have no willpower.
  ☐ Never ☐ Rarely ☐ Sometimes ☐ Often ☐ Always

- I already "cheated."
  ☐ Never ☐ Rarely ☐ Sometimes ☐ Often ☐ Always

Dieters have an endless number of reasons (excuses) to eat more than they should. You'll learn to respond to these kinds of sabotaging thoughts by reminding yourself that you have a choice: You can give in to these excuses, eat too much, and never get (or stay) thinner; OR you can stick to your plan.

When you see food you know you really shouldn't eat, how often do you think, *It's okay to eat this food because* ...

- People will think I'm strange [if I eat differently from them].
  ☐ Never ☐ Rarely ☐ Sometimes ☐ Often ☐ Always

- If I don't eat it, I'll displease someone.
  ☐ Never ☐ Rarely ☐ Sometimes ☐ Often ☐ Always

- Someone told me not to.
  ☐ Never ☐ Rarely ☐ Sometimes ☐ Often ☐ Always

- Everyone else is eating it.
  ☐ Never ☐ Rarely ☐ Sometimes ☐ Often ☐ Always

It's interesting how dieters can justify overeating based on other people's attitudes and behavior. But it is just a rationalization. If you want to lose excess weight and keep it off, you have to consistently work toward this goal, no matter what other people say or do.

could you have an eating disorder?

Many people try diet after diet and have a hard time achieving or maintaining weight loss. If that's true for you, you've come to the right place. However, if you have an eating disorder, you need professional care. Please answer the following questions:

- Do you continually obsess about your weight to the exclusion of more important aspects of your life?

- Do you weigh in the lower range of your ideal weight? (If you don't know what your ideal weight should be, check with a health-care provider.)

- Do you have a history of severe food restriction?

- Do you binge-eat and purge or abuse laxatives?

- Do you significantly overexercise to keep your weight down?

If you answered yes to any of the questions above, the Beck Diet Solution program is not for you; please see a health-care professional for specialized treatment.

Now that you've finished the questionnaire, I'd like you to look over your answers and write down a few important things you've learned about yourself:

_____

_____

_____

_____

_____

_____

_____

_____

_____

_____

_____

_____

_____

_____

_____

chapter 4

How to Motivate Yourself

I'm sure you have many reasons to want to lose weight. You could probably rattle off about a dozen of them right now. However, if you're like most people who struggle with dieting, you don't automatically think of all of these reasons when you're triggered to eat something you shouldn't. One essential technique that helps you control your eating is to continually remind yourself of these reasons, even when you're *not* tempted, so you'll be motivated to stop yourself when you *are* tempted.

The chart on the facing page lists reasons I've compiled from dieters I've counseled over the years. Check off every reason that applies to you and then write in additional reasons you can think of. Keep adding to the list as time goes on and you discover other wonderful benefits that you're not aware of yet. You'll read this list many, many times in the days and weeks and months (and even years!) to come.

On the reverse side of this list, you'll find an inventory of common disadvantages of dieting along with helpful responses in bold. Review both lists whenever you're tempted to eat something you shouldn't or whenever you start to feel resentful or burdened by your dieting requirements. Look at this second chart on page 34 now and put a check mark next to each idea you find helpful.

When you've completed these two charts, you're ready to learn more about the Beck Diet Solution program.

Reasons I Want to Lose Weight Chart

Check off all of the advantages that apply to you. Use the additional blank spaces
to fill in others that are more specific to your life.

Advantages to Losing Weight	Advantages to Losing Weight
☐ I'll look better and more attractive.	
☐ I'll have more confidence.	
☐ I'll be able to wear a smaller size.	
☐ I'll fit into more fashionable clothing.	
☐ I'll be able to buy fancy new underwear.	
☐ I'll feel happier when I look in the mirror.	
☐ I'll enjoy trying on clothes.	
☐ I'll feel better in a bathing suit.	
☐ I won't feel so self-conscious.	
☐ I'll get more compliments.	
☐ My blood pressure will go down.	
☐ My cholesterol will be reduced.	
☐ I'll be at less risk to develop type 2 diabetes.	
☐ I'll feel better physically.	
☐ I'll have more stamina.	
☐ I'll have more energy.	
☐ I'll feel more optimistic.	
☐ I'll make a better impression on people.	
☐ I'll be able to keep up with my kids.	
☐ I'll be less inhibited about my body.	
☐ I'll enjoy physical intimacy more.	
☐ I'll like myself better.	
☐ I'll feel as if I have accomplished something important.	
☐ I'll be more willing to find a job or make other life changes.	
☐ I'll be less self-critical.	
☐ I'll do more things in public, such as dancing or swimming.	
☐ My family won't remark about my weight or my eating.	
☐ I'll be more assertive.	
☐ I'll be more comfortable eating in front of others.	
☐ I'll feel in control.	

Disadvantages of Dieting with Helpful Responses

I don't want to feel deprived ...

BUT I can modify my plan in advance to include my favorite foods. Besides, I'd rather tolerate some deprivation and be thinner than eat whatever I want—whenever I want—and be heavier.

I don't want to tolerate hunger and cravings ...

BUT there are a lot of things I can do to decrease my discomfort and if I don't learn how to get myself to tolerate some discomfort, I won't be able to maintain the weight I lose.

I don't want to have to eat differently from other people ...

BUT that's the price I need to pay sometimes to get thinner and stay thinner.

I don't want to write down a plan for what I'm going to eat; I want to eat spontaneously ...

BUT I can't do that and expect to maintain weight loss in the long term.

I don't want to have to change my routine to make time and energy for dieting ...

BUT I have to face the fact that I won't be successful unless I do so.

I don't want other people to be unhappy with me because of the changes I'm making ...

BUT I'm entitled to do what I need to do to lose weight, as long as I'm not maliciously doing something to make someone else feel bad.

The Program

The Basics

The Beck Diet Solution program lasts for six weeks. You'll learn important skills to get ready for dieting during the first two weeks. Then you'll actually start your diet at the beginning of the third week. For each day, read the day's entry, work on the tasks throughout the day, and then check them off as you finish. Each night, look at that day's to-do list. Check off the items you've completed and circle any uncompleted items so that you can face the fact that you're not doing everything you need to do to lose excess weight.

If you feel unmotivated, it's because sabotaging thoughts—ideas that pop into your head and undermine your resolve—are getting in the way. Read the perforated Response Cards at the back of this workbook and consider creating your own. The "helpful responses" above each to-do list may be useful as a basis for creating additional cards. If you're *still* having difficulty motivating yourself, call your diet coach.

Starting on Day 14 (page 79), you'll fill in My Daily Food Plan Chart so you can decide in advance what you're going to eat each day and then monitor your food intake. You'll continue to do this for the last four weeks of the program. In addition, after Day 42 (page 241), you'll print out blank charts and graphs to help you continue losing weight or transition from dieting to maintenance.

You'll need to gather a few items in addition to this workbook. Check them off as you get them:

☐ **Sticky notes** for marking pages in the workbook that you want to access easily so you can look at them often; for "tabbing" the weight graph and day you are currently working on; and for writing reminder notes that you can post in such places as your bathroom mirror, computer, and refrigerator door.

☐ **Cardstock paper** to make additional Response Cards that are the same size as the perforated ones in the back of the workbook. Or you can cut index cards, file folders, or cards to size, if you prefer.

☐ **A food scale** and measuring cups and spoons

☐ **A bathroom scale**

Make the program work for you. Can you complete more than one day's tasks at a time? Sure, go as fast as you'd like—*as long as you do every task.* Can you go much slower? Again, the answer is yes. Go at your own pace.

On the other hand, if you've already started dieting or are trying to maintain weight loss, can you skip some steps? No, please don't skip any and be sure to complete all of the steps in order. Even though you might not need to use all of the techniques at this point, you'll need to implement them at some time in the future. I want you to learn these skills now so you'll be fully equipped for the more difficult times. Do all of the tasks in this workbook. They are essential for long-term success.

One last thing: You'll notice that the word *cheat* is not used in the rest of the workbook. I don't like the term *cheating* because it is likely to demoralize you and may lead you to view yourself as "bad." And if you're like many chronic dieters, somehow using the word gives you license to abandon your diet for the rest of the day: *I cheated ... I shouldn't have had those French fries ... I may as well [eat whatever I want today and] start again tomorrow.* For some dieters with this attitude, tomorrow never comes and they just keep eating—and gaining. I prefer the term *mistake.* It helps reinforce that even if you eat something that isn't on your diet, it doesn't mean that the rest of the day is ruined. You're only human; you made a mistake. But you can get right back on track.

Now, you're ready to begin!

chapter 5

Week 1

Create a Foundation for Diet Success

As you start this first week, I hope you're excited and have begun to see how Cognitive Therapy techniques will enable you to lose excess weight and keep it off—*permanently.* But don't rush into dieting just yet! In order to be successful this time, you need to learn and practice such skills as tolerating hunger and resisting cravings. Even if you don't need these skills today, you're going to need them when you hit your first difficult day—and I want you to know precisely what to do *before* you get to that point. It is crucial to spend time now learning techniques you'll use for the rest of your life whenever the going gets tough. That's why this week's theme is "create a foundation for diet success."

If you still want to start dieting this minute, think of it this way: Getting ready to diet is like training for a marathon. You wouldn't just sign up today and run a 25-mile race tomorrow. You need to do lots of practice runs to build up your strength and stamina. Without training and practice, you're likely to become discouraged and drop out of the race. Dieting is similar—you have to "train," building up your diet muscles and stamina—so that you can finish the race and win.

day 1

Review the Advantages of Dieting

I t's crucial for you to rehearse again and again all of the reasons you want to lose weight so that they'll feel compelling when you are driven to have that second serving or to grab an unplanned snack. Check off each task below as you accomplish it:

☐ Turn to the list of reasons you have for losing weight on page 33. Cut out the page along the dotted lines.

☐ Make at least one additional copy of the list so that you will have one to carry with you wherever you go and one (or more) to post where you are most likely to see it.

☐ Notice that the reverse side of the page contains helpful responses to a list of dieting disadvantages. Decide whether you want to copy and post these responses as well.

☐ Be creative in making extra lists. For example, photocopy the list on colored paper to make it distinctive. Copy the reasons that are most important to you on a 3 x 5 index card or inside a pretty, blank greeting card. Or use your computer to create a card or to make a screen saver for yourself. If you're "wired," program your e-mail, cell phone, or personal digital assistant (PDA) to send this list to you a few times a day.

☐ Post the list where you'll easily see it: Put it on your bathroom or bedroom mirror or on your refrigerator or kitchen cabinet. Or tape the list to one of the inside or outside covers of this workbook.

☐ Make sure to take a copy of the list with you in your wallet, purse, or pocket so that you'll have it whenever you need it.

☐ Decide exactly when you plan to read the list. For the next two weeks, I'd like you to read it at least once a day. When you actually start dieting, you should read it more often. You might find it helpful to read it right before every meal, for example. You should also definitely schedule yourself to read it at your trigger times—those moments during the day when you're likely to succumb to cravings.

☐ If you think you may have trouble remembering to read your list at times, set up a reminder system for yourself (post a sticky note or set an alarm, for example).

☐ If you have sabotaging thoughts that get in the way of doing this assignment, tear out Response Card #1 ("Do It Anyway") from the back of the workbook. Read it as often as necessary. Also copy onto a card the helpful response on the next page if you think you'll benefit from reading it.

what are you thinking?

Sabotaging Thought: Losing weight is very important to me. I'm always aware of why I want to do it, so I don't need to read the list.

Helpful Response: When I'm craving, my mind is focused on getting food, not on getting thinner. That's why I have to cement the reasons in my mind by reading the list every day.

today's to-do list

Each night, remember to check off each task you've completed. Circle any task you didn't complete so you can face the fact that you didn't do everything you need to do to lose weight and keep it off. Remember, *not* doing all of these tasks in the past didn't lead to lasting weight loss and all its benefits.

☐ I read my list of reasons to lose weight at least once today.

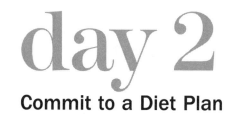

day 2
Commit to a Diet Plan

I n Chapter 2 of this workbook, I asked you to consider what kind of diet you wanted to try. If needed, review pages 21–24. Check with your health-care professional to make sure the diet is suitable for you. Then do the following:

☐ Choose a primary diet *and* a backup diet, in case the initial diet plan isn't working for you. Make sure the diets meet all of the criteria on page 24.

Primary:_____   Backup:_____

☐ Reread page 23 to help you figure out whether you should modify the diet so you can stay on it, no matter the circumstances. Remember that it's important to *plan modifications in advance*. I don't want you to get in the habit of making decisions on the spot to deviate from your diet. I have found that *last-minute deviations are a primary reason dieters regain lost weight*.

☐ Do not modify your diet in these ways: skipping breakfast, eating less than your diet calls for to lose weight more quickly, and being strict on weekdays but "loose" on weekends. Research shows that doing any of these things invariably leads to weight gain. Write your modifications here:

_____

_____

what are you thinking?

Sabotaging Thought: Some diets must be better than others. The media is full of diets that say you can lose weight quickly and easily—and still eat anything you want!

Helpful Response: No scientific research supports there is a "magic" diet, pill, or supplement. If I want to lose weight, I have to consume fewer calories than I expend.

today's to-do list

Each night, remember to check off each task you've completed. Circle any you should have completed but didn't, so you can be aware that you didn't follow the program completely.

☐ I read my list of reasons to lose weight.

date: _____

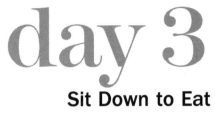

Sit Down to Eat

On Day 15 (page 85), you'll begin restricting your eating. So now it's very important for you to learn how to notice and savor every bite you eat. Since it's hard to do this when you're standing up or walking around, you usually end up eating too much, either at the time or later on. Before you begin your diet, I want you to master the skill of eating while sitting. Here are your tasks for the day:

☐ Starting today, eat 100 percent of your food while sitting down.

☐ If you feel resistant at any point, ask yourself what's going through your mind. Are you having any of the following sabotaging thoughts?

- *I'm too busy to sit down.*

- *It's okay because I have to taste what I'm cooking.*

- *If I don't eat the leftovers as I'm clearing the table, they'll just go to waste.*

- *I'm just having a little bite; it's not really a meal.*

- *Other people are standing up and eating (at a party, fair, food store, etc.), so it's okay if I do, too.*

☐ Write down any other sabotaging thoughts you have: _____

_____

_____

_____

_____

☐ Whenever you have a sabotaging thought that undermines your motivation to eat sitting down, read your list of reasons to lose weight as well as Response Card #1 ("Do It Anyway") from the back of this workbook.

☐ Make your own Response Cards. You can use the helpful responses on the facing page as models, if they're applicable.

what are you thinking?

Sabotaging Thought: I don't have time to sit down for every meal and snack.

Helpful Response: Standing up is not an option—I have NO CHOICE. I will have to rearrange my schedule so that I *do* have time if I want to lose weight and keep it off.

Sabotaging Thought: I'll eat standing up just this one time.

Helpful Response: "Just this once" has a tendency to turn into "way too often." I have to develop a lifetime skill of making myself sit down while eating if I want a lifetime of being thinner.

today's to-do list

Each night, remember to check off each task you've completed. Circle any you didn't do, so you can be aware that you didn't follow the program completely.

☐ I read my list of reasons to lose weight (and other Response Cards as needed).

☐ I ate everything while sitting down.

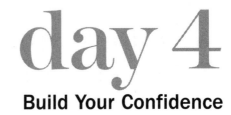

day 4

Build Your Confidence

One of the biggest problems dieters face is a sense of helplessness when they stray from their diet or when the number on the scale fails to go down. They often have sabotaging thoughts, such as, *Oh, no, I thought I could do this! I thought I could lose weight! But I was wrong.*

You need to start building a sense of confidence that you can do what you have to do to lose weight. That's why I want you to start giving yourself credit for every positive eating behavior you engage in and every helpful eating decision you make *starting right now* so that you can develop this important habit.

Check off each item below as you complete it:

☐ Tear out and read Response Card #2 ("Give Myself Credit"). Carry it around with you to develop this habit.

☐ Think what you would say to your best friend if she did something that you thought she deserved credit for. You'd probably say something along these lines: "You did it!" "That's really good!" "Great!" "You deserve credit." "Good job." Whatever you would say to her is what I want you to say to yourself.

☐ Put a rubber band or special bracelet around your wrist. Throughout the day, whenever you notice you're wearing it, the bracelet will remind you to give yourself credit.

☐ Give yourself credit every time you make a check mark on one of your to-do lists.

☐ Write down in the daily to-do lists other diet-related creditworthy things you do. For example, even though you haven't officially started your diet, were there any times today that you served yourself a smaller portion than usual, chose a lower-calorie food, refrained from taking a second helping, resisted the temptation to eat between meals, or tolerated feeling hungry?

☐ Watch out for self-criticism that undermines your confidence. When you eat something you shouldn't or skip an exercise session, think about what you'd say to your best friend if she made the same mistake.

☐ Answer back any sabotaging thoughts you have about this assignment and make Response Cards if you think they'll help. Read examples of helpful responses on the facing page.

what are you thinking?

Sabotaging Thought: I haven't really done anything that difficult so far.

Helpful Response: It doesn't matter whether the changes I make are easy or difficult. I need to get in the habit of giving myself credit to build up my sense of effectiveness and control.

Sabotaging Thought: It's seems silly to praise myself—like getting a star on my paper when I was in grade school.

Helpful Response: It's not childish; it's absolutely essential to my success to recognize my achievements. Not giving myself credit in the past didn't lead to permanent weight loss.

today's to-do list

Each night, remember to check off each task you've completed. Circle any you didn't do, so you can be aware that you didn't follow the program completely.

☐ I read my list of reasons to lose weight (and other Response Cards as needed).

☐ I ate everything while sitting down.

☐ I gave myself credit for these things and for: _____

_____

_____

_____

_____

_____.

day 5

Slow Down and Be Mindful

Your next task is to improve your ability to enjoy every bite of food you eat, maximizing your psychological satisfaction by eating slowly and paying full attention to your food. If you eat too quickly, not only will you feel dissatisfied but also your food will be gone before your body has time to recognize that it's full. This feeling of fullness can take up to 20 minutes to register!

Here's what you should do: Eat alone at a dining table for breakfast and lunch today. Make sure you have no distractions, such as the TV, a book, the computer, or other people's conversation. Serve yourself your whole meal and take the serving dishes off the table before you begin eating. Then do the following tasks:

☐ Take small bites and chew slowly.

☐ Finish chewing and swallowing each bite before you put more food on your fork.

☐ Put your utensils down between every few bites and then count to 10 before you pick them up again.

☐ Take a sip of water every minute or two.

☐ If you're tempted to skip learning this skill, read Response Cards #1 ("Do It Anyway") and #3 ("Eat Mindfully").

In an ideal world, you'd never eat with distractions, but that's not realistic. If you're not watching TV, reading, or using the computer while you eat, it's probably because you're eating with other people. In any case, I want you to teach yourself how to focus your attention on every bite while also focusing on something else. So at dinner tonight, do the following:

☐ To remind yourself to use all of the slow-down techniques above, change something in your environment. Put a sticky note by your place setting. Use different flatware or dishes. Or set a timer to go off every couple of minutes.

what are you thinking?

Sabotaging Thought: It feels unnatural to make myself eat slowly.

Helpful Response: The more I practice, the more natural it will become. It's an essential skill.

today's to-do list

Each night, remember to check off each task you've completed. Circle any you didn't do, so you can be aware that you didn't follow the program completely.

☐ I read my list of reasons to lose weight (and other Response Cards as needed).

☐ I ate everything slowly and mindfully while sitting down.

☐ I gave myself credit for these things and for: _____

_____

_____

_____

_____

_____.

day 6

Meet with Your Diet Coach

Today is the day you should talk (in person or on the phone) to the diet coach you selected before starting the program, as I described on pages 20–21 of this workbook. Do the following:

☐ Set a definite "appointment" to talk to him/her at a specific time, once a week (preferably in person) on the days you're going to record your change in weight (days 15, 22, 29, 36, and so on).

☐ Figure out a system to contact your coach at other times. Discuss the possibility of talking by phone at the start and/or end of every weekend, since these are vulnerable times for most people.

☐ In the beginning—or when you're going through a rough period—consider having daily contact with your coach. For example, you could e-mail or leave voice-mail messages telling how you're doing. Having even a small difficulty can be a signal for your coach to contact you.

Whatever plan you settle on, be sure to make it explicit and official. Once you start dieting, discuss the following with your coach during your weekly appointments:

• Weight change, plus or minus

• Successes and accomplishments in both dieting and exercise

• Problems you had since you talked last (what sabotaging thoughts you had, what you did in response, what you could say to yourself and do the next time this kind of situation occurs)

• Situations you think might arise before you talk next, such as going to a party (ask your coach to help you do some advance problem solving)

If you're tempted to skip this assignment, read Response Card #1 ("Do It Anyway") and see if the sabotaging thought and helpful response on the facing page are applicable.

what are you thinking?

Sabotaging Thought: I can do this on my own.

Helpful Response: It's a million times more likely that *this* time I'll be able to lose weight and keep it off if I have to report to my coach and get help when I need it.

today's to-do list

Each night, remember to check off each task you've completed. Circle any you didn't do, so you can be aware that you didn't follow the program completely.

☐ I read my list of reasons to lose weight (and other Response Cards as needed).

☐ I ate everything slowly and mindfully while sitting down.

☐ I talked to my diet coach and devised the following plan: _____

_____

_____

_____

☐ I gave myself credit for these things and for: _____

_____

_____

_____

_____

date: _____

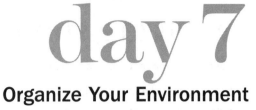

Organize Your Environment

It's difficult to stick to your diet when tempting foods you're not supposed to have are too easily accessible in your kitchen or at work. Later on, it will get easier and you'll be able to keep most foods around. But in the beginning of your diet, it's important to get rid of items that you find difficult to resist and to stock your kitchen with healthy foods you *can* eat. Do the following now to prepare for starting your diet:

☐ Develop an attitude of entitlement. Losing weight is very important to you, and you deserve to have your family make reasonable accommodations (if relevant). Read Response Card #4 ("It's Okay to Disappoint People").

☐ Discuss with your diet coach what you should ask your family to do and what you can say to them to get their cooperation. For example, perhaps they could buy only a single-serving size, instead of a larger portion, of foods that are particularly hard for you to resist.

☐ Go through your kitchen and put on the counter any tempting foods that aren't on your diet. Then either give them away or throw them away.

☐ If you have trouble, read Response Card #5 ("Say No to Extra Food").

Preparing your work environment may be more challenging, since you can't always avoid the foods that are there. Here are some changes you *can* make (and you don't have to tell anyone you're on a diet if you don't want to—you can just say that you've decided to start eating in a more healthy way):

☐ If you bring lunch or a snack with you, keep it out of sight until it's time to eat it.

☐ Ask coworkers who bring food for general consumption to the office kitchen if you can put it in a cabinet and post a note telling everyone where the food is.

☐ Ask your cafeteria to include healthier options, if they don't already.

☐ Make a deal with yourself: If there are some highly tempting foods that you hadn't planned to eat available at work, wrap up a small piece and take it home. Plan to eat it the next day. (Of course, you'll need to plan to eat less of some other food that day.)

what are you thinking?

Sabotaging Thought: I don't want to ask others to make changes.

Helpful Response: At the beginning, I have to minimize food triggers. And it's good practice for me to stand up for myself.

today's to-do list

Each night, remember to check off each task you've completed. Circle any you didn't do, so you can be aware that you didn't follow the program completely.

☐ I read my list of reasons to lose weight (and other Response Cards as needed).

☐ I ate everything slowly and mindfully while sitting down.

☐ I arranged my work and home environments to meet my diet needs.

☐ I gave myself credit for these things and for: _____

_____

_____

_____

_____

_____.

Week 2

Get Ready for Dieting

Was last week different from what you expected? Did you know how much there was to learn just to get ready for dieting? Well, there's more, which is why I don't suggest that you start your diet quite yet. This week, you're going to learn two basic skills. You're going to learn how to schedule in time for dieting and exercise activities. A major reason dieters regain weight is that they stop taking the time they need to do these things. Another major reason dieters regain excess weight is that they have never learned to tolerate hunger and cravings. This week, you'll do exercises to prove to yourself that you *can* stand hunger and cravings and that they come and go.

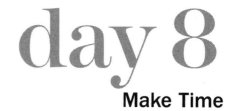

day 8

Make Time

I wish I could tell you that you could easily lose weight—and keep it off—without having to change your schedule. But that's not realistic. Losing weight takes time and energy. You're going to have to develop a new mindset: *Losing weight is so important to me that I'm willing to fit my life around the necessary activities* (instead of vice versa). Here's what you're going to need time for this week:

- Exercising for a minimum of 30 minutes three times a week

- Engaging in brief daily exercise

- Continuing to work in this workbook

- Continuing to sit down and eat every meal and snack slowly and mindfully

☐ Look at the Sample Daily Schedule on page 54. Then write in all the diet and exercise activities you need to do today on My Daily Schedule on page 55. If you like, you can also use this chart to write in the rest of your activities for the day.

You'll continue to fill out a daily schedule each morning throughout the program. Starting next week, you'll add in more diet-related activities:

- Shopping for food on your diet plan, as often as necessary

- Taking extra time to prepare meals, if necessary

☐ Every evening this week, ask yourself, *When would I have been able to do these extra diet-related activities today?*

If you have difficulty figuring out how to make time, think about what you do in the course of a normal day:

☐ List each activity, according to its importance (Essential, Highly Desirable, and Desirable), on My Priority Chart on page 57. (Use the Sample Priority Chart on page 56 as an example.)

☐ Meet with your diet coach. Look at each activity and decide which ones you can postpone, eliminate, cut back on, or delegate.

☐ Start reading Response Card #6 ("Put Dieting First") every day.

Sample Daily Schedule

(A typical weekday)

Time	Activity
6:00 a.m.	
6:30	
7:00	Eat breakfast slowly.
7:30	
8:00	Read diet workbook.
8:30	
9:00	Park at far end of parking lot at work.
9:30	
10:00	
10:30	
11:00	
11:30	
Noon	Take stairs down and walk to coffee shop.
12:30 p.m.	Eat lunch slowly, walk back, and take stairs up.
1:00	
1:30	
2:00	
2:30	
3:00	Take 5-minute walk around building.
3:30	
4:00	
4:30	
5:00	
5:30	Go to gym. Park 1 block away.
6:00	
6:30	
7:00	Eat dinner slowly.
7:30	
8:00	
8:30	
9:00	Fill out to-do list.
9:30	
10:00	
10:30	
11:00	

My Daily Schedule

Use this chart to plan your diet and exercise activities for today. If you work the night shift or follow a routine that is different from the one noted here, write in times that are appropriate to your situation.

Time	Activity
6:00 a.m.	
6:30	
7:00	
7:30	
8:00	
8:30	
9:00	
9:30	
10:00	
10:30	
11:00	
11:30	
Noon	
12:30 p.m.	
1:00	
1:30	
2:00	
2:30	
3:00	
3:30	
4:00	
4:30	
5:00	
5:30	
6:00	
6:30	
7:00	
7:30	
8:00	
8:30	
9:00	
9:30	
10:00	
10:30	
11:00	

Sample Priority Chart

Essential Activities	Highly Desirable	Desirable
Personal-care activities	Organize papers.	Fix up apartment.
Work	Take dog for longer walks.	Join book club.
Walk dog.	Additional household chores	Additional time surfing the Internet
Household chores (clean up; dishes; bills; laundry)	Work in garden.	Additional time reading
Food shopping and meal preparation	Plan a vacation.	Manicures
Visit grandmother.	More personal time (computer games; reading newspaper)	Lower-priority errands
Some errands	Clothes shopping	Entertaining
Personal e-mails and phone calls	Spend additional time with friends/family.	Movies, plays, museums, etc.
Spiritual activities	Babysit for nephew.	Watch other TV shows.
Visit friends/family.	Watch favorite TV show.	
Doctor appointments	Volunteer work	

My Priority Chart

Essential Activities	Highly Desirable	Desirable

what are you thinking?

Sabotaging Thought: I'd rather just see how things go, instead of planning.

Helpful Response: I have to learn the skill of scheduling now in preparation for more hectic times.

today's to-do list

Each night, remember to check off each task you've completed. Circle any you didn't do, so you can be aware that you didn't follow the program completely.

☐ I read my list of reasons to lose weight (and other Response Cards as needed).

☐ I scheduled exercise and dieting activities on My Daily Schedule.

☐ I ate everything slowly and mindfully while sitting down.

☐ I prioritized my activities.

☐ I gave myself credit for these things and for: _____

_____

_____

_____

_____

_____ .

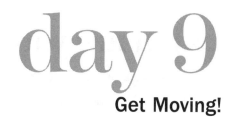

day 9

Get Moving!

Have you picked an exercise program yet? If not, review page 25. Remember, the goal is to work up to at least 30 minutes of exercise three times a week, with a brief period of exercise daily. Even a five-minute walk is better than no walk at all. You're also going to fit in as much spontaneous exercise as you can by taking the stairs, walking to your destination, and so on.

Commit in writing to make exercise a priority:

My exercise program will be: _____

_____

_____

_____

_____.

Here is a list of things for you to do:

☐ Check with your health-care professional before you start any exercise program.

☐ Give yourself credit every time you exercise.

☐ Be accountable to your diet coach. Call (you can leave a voice-mail message) or e-mail daily about your exercise until the habit is strongly entrenched.

☐ Set realistic exercise goals. Start small and build up a little more each week.

☐ Resist exercise saboteurs (yourself or other people) who tell you that other things are more important than exercise. Read Response Card #7 ("Exercise No Matter What") every day to help motivate yourself.

☐ Write down when you're going to exercise (even if it's just for as little as five minutes) on your daily schedule.

what are you thinking?

Sabotaging Thought: If I can't exercise for 30 minutes, it's not worth exercising at all.

Helpful Response: Five minutes is better than zero minutes, and it's essential for me not to break my exercise *habit.*

today's to-do list

Each night, remember to check off each task you've completed. Circle any you didn't do, so you can be aware that you didn't follow the program completely.

☐ I read my list of reasons to lose weight (and other Response Cards as needed).

☐ I scheduled exercise and dieting activities on My Daily Schedule.

☐ I ate everything slowly and mindfully while sitting down.

☐ I gave myself credit for these things and for: _____

_____

_____

_____

_____

_____.

My Daily Schedule

Use this chart to plan your diet and exercise activities for today.

Time	Activity
6:00 a.m.	
6:30	
7:00	
7:30	
8:00	
8:30	
9:00	
9:30	
10:00	
10:30	
11:00	
11:30	
Noon	
12:30 p.m.	
1:00	
1:30	
2:00	
2:30	
3:00	
3:30	
4:00	
4:30	
5:00	
5:30	
6:00	
6:30	
7:00	
7:30	
8:00	
8:30	
9:00	
9:30	
10:00	
10:30	
11:00	

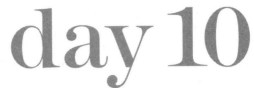

day 10

Set Achievable Goals

A weight-loss goal can initially make you feel excited, hopeful, and motivated. But if it begins to feel too difficult or too far away from being achieved, you can begin to feel overwhelmed or discouraged. Here are your tasks for today:

☐ Do not set an ultimate goal. Instead, set a goal to lose 5 pounds.

☐ Plan how you're going to celebrate when you lose 5 pounds. Give yourself lots of credit, celebrate with your coach, and reward yourself in some non-food-related way. For example, treat yourself to tickets to a concert.

After you reach your first 5-pound weight-loss goal, then set a new goal to lose 5 more pounds—and so on and so on. You'll find blank weight-loss graphs at Day 22 (page 127) and at Day 42 (page 246) to help you keep track of your losses. And, remember, *slow* weight loss is healthy and more likely to be long lasting.

what are you thinking?

Sabotaging Thought: I'm not going to be satisfied until I get to my ultimate goal.

Helpful Response: My ultimate goal may or may not be realistic and is probably far off. I should work toward being happy every time I lose 5 pounds.

today's to-do list

Each night, remember to check off each task you've completed. Circle any you didn't do, so you can be aware that you didn't follow the program completely.

☐ I read my list of reasons to lose weight (and other Response Cards as needed).

☐ I scheduled exercise and dieting activities on My Daily Schedule.

☐ I ate everything slowly and mindfully while sitting down.

☐ I exercised (for at least 5 to 30 minutes).

☐ I decided on the following plan to reward myself when I lose 5 pounds: _____

_____

_____

☐ I gave myself credit for these things and for: _____

_____

_____

_____

_____

_____.

My Daily Schedule

Use this chart to plan your diet and exercise activities for today.

Time	Activity
6:00 a.m.	
6:30	
7:00	
7:30	
8:00	
8:30	
9:00	
9:30	
10:00	
10:30	
11:00	
11:30	
Noon	
12:30 p.m.	
1:00	
1:30	
2:00	
2:30	
3:00	
3:30	
4:00	
4:30	
5:00	
5:30	
6:00	
6:30	
7:00	
7:30	
8:00	
8:30	
9:00	
9:30	
10:00	
10:30	
11:00	

day 11

date: _____

Learn the Difference Between Hunger, Desire, and Cravings

Today, you're going to learn a very important skill: being able to tell the difference between just wanting to eat, actually being hungry, and having a craving. Discover how to do this by practicing the following:

☐ Every hour on the hour, wherever you are, whatever you're doing, until you go to bed at night, ask yourself, *Do I feel like eating now?*

☐ If the answer is yes, notice what's going on in your mouth, throat, and body. Then ask yourself the following questions to label your experience and note it on page 66:

☐ Has it been at least a couple of hours since you last ate, does your stomach feel empty, and could you feel satisfied if you ate a range of foods? If so, you are probably hungry.

☐ Does your stomach feel reasonably comfortable, but you just *feel* like eating? If so, that's probably a desire.

☐ Do you have a strong urge to eat a particular food or kind of food, with a yearning in your mouth, throat, or body? If so, that's probably a craving.

One dieter I counseled found this exercise very helpful. (See her partially filled-out chart below.) Not only did she realize that she had been labeling any desire or urge to eat as hunger, but also she found that her cravings and hunger came and went—they didn't just get worse.

Sample Monitoring Chart

Time	Sensations	Label (hunger, desire, craving)
1:00 p.m.	none	none
2:00	slight desire in mouth (for chips in vending machine)	desire
3:00	none	none
4:00	strong urge, yearning in mouth (for chips)	craving
5:00	none	none
6:00	emptiness and rumbling in stomach	hunger

After completing this exercise, you, too, should be in a much better position to distinguish between hunger, desire, and cravings. Repeat this exercise as often as necessary, until you no longer have difficulty differentiating between these three states.

Time	Sensations	Label (hunger, desire, craving)
My Monitoring Chart		
7:00 a.m.		
8:00		
9:00		
10:00		
11:00		
Noon		
1:00 p.m.		
2:00		
3:00		
4:00		
5:00		
6:00		
7:00		
8:00		
9:00		
10:00		
11:00		

what are you thinking?

Sabotaging Thought: I know when I'm hungry and when I'm not. I don't need to fill out a chart.

Helpful Response: Chances are, I sometimes have a desire or craving but label it as hunger—which gives me an excuse to eat. Monitoring the difference today on a chart will make it more likely that I won't be able to use this excuse in the future and end up gaining weight.

today's to-do list

Each night, remember to check off each task you've completed. Circle any you didn't do, so you can be aware that you didn't follow the program completely.

☐ I read my list of reasons to lose weight (and other Response Cards as needed).

☐ I scheduled exercise and dieting activities on My Daily Schedule.

☐ I ate everything slowly and mindfully while sitting down.

☐ I exercised (for at least 5 to 30 minutes).

☐ I filled out My Monitoring Chart to distinguish hunger from desire and cravings.

☐ I gave myself credit for these things and for: _____

_____

_____

_____

_____

_____ .

My Daily Schedule

Use this chart to plan your diet and exercise activities for today.

Time	Activity
6:00 a.m.	
6:30	
7:00	
7:30	
8:00	
8:30	
9:00	
9:30	
10:00	
10:30	
11:00	
11:30	
Noon	
12:30 p.m.	
1:00	
1:30	
2:00	
2:30	
3:00	
3:30	
4:00	
4:30	
5:00	
5:30	
6:00	
6:30	
7:00	
7:30	
8:00	
8:30	
9:00	
9:30	
10:00	
10:30	
11:00	

day 12

Prove You Can Tolerate Hunger and Cravings

Learning to refrain from eating when it's not yet time for you to eat is a key aspect of successful dieting. Every time you refrain, you build up your "resistance habit." Every time you end up eating, you build up your "giving-in habit." If you have the sabotaging thought, *I'm hungry, so I have to eat,* it's important to recognize that while it's true you feel uncomfortable, it is *not* true that you *have* to eat.

I'd like you to recognize that hunger and cravings are uncomfortable, but not nearly as uncomfortable as other experiences you've tolerated in your life. To learn this, do the following:

☐ Think back to the worst discomfort you've ever felt. Label that experience and write it next to "Severe Discomfort" on My Discomfort Scale below. (Follow the example in the Sample Discomfort Scale.)

☐ Do the same for an experience that was only moderately uncomfortable and one that was mildly uncomfortable.

Sample Discomfort Scale

Severity	Experience
severe discomfort	when I broke my arm
moderate discomfort	when I had a really bad backache
mild discomfort	when I had a headache

My Discomfort Scale

Severity	Experience
severe discomfort	_____
moderate discomfort	_____
mild discomfort	_____

Today, I'd like you to eat breakfast and then not eat again until dinner (check with your health-care professional first if you have a medical condition that could prevent you from safely doing so). Doing this is the best way for you to prove to yourself that hunger and cravings aren't "bad," that they come and go, that they are *never an emergency,* and that you, therefore, never *have* to respond by eating. Every hour on the hour, do the following:

☐ Rate how uncomfortable your sensations of hunger and craving are (none, mild, moderate, or severe) on My Discomfort Chart on the facing page. (Use the Sample Discomfort Chart below as an example.)

☐ Reflect on the preceding hour and record the range of discomfort you experienced.

Sample Discomfort Chart

Time	Discomfort at the Moment	Range of Discomfort in the Past Hour (none, mild, moderate, or severe)
6:00 a.m.	asleep	--------------
7:00	none	none
8:00	none	none
9:00	none	none to mild
10:00	mild	none to mild
11:00	none	none to mild
Noon	mild	none to mild
1:00 p.m.	none	none to mild
2:00	mild	none to mild
3:00	mild	none to mild
4:00	none	none to mild
5:00	mild	none to mild
6:00	mild	none to mild
7:00	none	none
8:00	none	none
9:00	none	none to mild
10:00	mild	none to mild
11:00	none	none

I think you'll find the same thing as the dieter who filled out the Sample Discomfort Scale when she skipped lunch: Compared with a broken arm and a bad backache, even her *worst* hunger and cravings were only mildly uncomfortable. She was also surprised to find that even when intensely hungry, she didn't stay that way for a full hour. In fact, the hunger usually lasted about 15 minutes—then disappeared.

My Discomfort Chart

Time	Discomfort at the Moment	Range of Discomfort in the Past Hour (none, mild, moderate, or severe)
6:00 a.m.		
7:00		
8:00		
9:00		
10:00		
11:00		
Noon		
1:00 p.m.		
2:00		
3:00		
4:00		
5:00		
6:00		
7:00		
8:00		
9:00		
10:00		
11:00		

what are you thinking?

Sabotaging Thought: I'm so hungry. Shouldn't I be able to eat?

Helpful Response: It's good that I'm feeling hungry! People without weight problems feel hungry every day—they just don't think much about it. They just wait until their next meal to satisfy that hunger. Tolerating hunger (and cravings) is an essential skill to losing weight and then maintaining a healthy weight for my whole life.

today's to-do list

Each night, remember to check off each task you've completed. Circle any you didn't do, so you can be aware that you didn't follow the program completely.

☐ I read my list of reasons to lose weight (and other Response Cards as needed).

☐ I scheduled exercise and dieting activities on My Daily Schedule.

☐ I ate everything slowly and mindfully while sitting down.

☐ I exercised (for at least 5 to 30 minutes).

☐ I filled out My Discomfort Scale and My Discomfort Chart.

☐ I gave myself credit for these things and for: _____

_____

_____

_____

_____

_____ .

My Daily Schedule

Use this chart to plan your diet and exercise activities for today.

Time	Activity
6:00 a.m.	
6:30	
7:00	
7:30	
8:00	
8:30	
9:00	
9:30	
10:00	
10:30	
11:00	
11:30	
Noon	
12:30 p.m.	
1:00	
1:30	
2:00	
2:30	
3:00	
3:30	
4:00	
4:30	
5:00	
5:30	
6:00	
6:30	
7:00	
7:30	
8:00	
8:30	
9:00	
9:30	
10:00	
10:30	
11:00	

day 13

Decrease Hunger and Cravings

Yesterday, you proved to yourself that hunger and cravings are uncomfortable but that you don't *have* to do anything about them. If you've learned that lesson, you can now work on reducing these uncomfortable states by turning your attention away from how you're feeling and toward something else. Try the following:

☐ Look at My Distraction Techniques Chart on pages 76–77 and add anything else you can think of that would let you turn your attention away from eating.

☐ Skip or postpone a meal or snacks today so that you can practice using these activities. Each time you find that you're hungry or having a craving, choose at least five activities to try. (You don't have to do all five if your hunger and cravings go away quickly.)

☐ When you finish each activity, rate how effective it was at reducing your discomfort.

☐ The next time you really want to eat something you shouldn't, select another five activities and rate them—and so on.

☐ Plan to try new activities in the days to come.

☐ Buy or gather whatever items you'll need to do the activities on the list and put these things in a special box: for example, a magazine, a needlepoint project, a DVD, a list of Web sites you've always wanted to look at, a computer game, a relaxation tape, a puzzle, nail polish, a list of friends/family to call. Make this list now:

I will get: _____

_____

_____

_____

_____.

☐ When you've discovered which techniques work best for you, add them to Response Card #9 ("Distraction Techniques").

what are you thinking?

Sabotaging Thought: I know I should get involved with other activities and refrain from eating this, but I just don't care.

Helpful Response: It's true that I don't care at this moment, but pretty soon I'm going to feel really bad that I ate this. When I get on the scale on Day 15 (page 85), I'm going to care very much. If I don't learn to resist eating food I'm not supposed to have, I'll never be able to keep off the weight I lose.

today's to-do list

Each night, remember to check off each task you've completed. Circle any you didn't do, so you can be aware that you didn't follow the program completely.

☐ I read my list of reasons to lose weight (and other Response Cards as needed).

☐ I scheduled exercise and dieting activities on My Daily Schedule.

☐ I ate everything slowly and mindfully while sitting down.

☐ I exercised (for at least 5 to 30 minutes).

☐ I skipped a meal or snack today and used distraction techniques.

☐ I gave myself credit for these things and for: _____

_____

_____

_____

_____

_____.

My Distraction Techniques Chart

Try up to five activities at a time when you're hungry or craving and rate how effective each one is.

Activity	Effectiveness (not at all, mild, moderate, very)
Read my list of reasons to lose weight.	
Read Response Cards.	
Read this workbook.	
Read another diet book.	
Look up diet Web sites.	
Phone my diet coach.	
Drink a no- or low-calorie beverage.	
Distance myself from food.	
Throw away food or move it.	
Play a computer game.	
Get out of the house.	
Listen to a relaxation tape.	
Practice an instrument.	
Do a jigsaw puzzle.	
Make a scrapbook.	
Organize my closet.	
Clean out my drawers.	
Go to the gym.	
Leaf through a catalog.	
Brush my teeth.	
Polish my nails.	
Call a friend or family member to chat.	
Take a walk.	
Ride a bike.	
Surf the Web.	
"Window-shop" via the Internet.	
Write e-mails or cards.	
Ride the elevator down and walk back up.	

My Distraction Techniques Chart

(continued)

Activity	Effectiveness (not at all, mild, moderate, very)
Take a bath or shower.	_____
Do a home-improvement project.	_____
Do a crafts project.	_____
Work in the garden.	_____
Make homemade or computer greeting cards.	_____
Download music.	_____
Read a magazine or book.	_____
Brush my pet.	_____
Do a puzzle in the newspaper.	_____
Plan a trip (real or fantasy).	_____
_____	_____
_____	_____
_____	_____
_____	_____
_____	_____
_____	_____
_____	_____
_____	_____
_____	_____
_____	_____
_____	_____
_____	_____

My Daily Schedule

Use this chart to plan your diet and exercise activities for today.

Time	Activity
6:00 a.m.	
6:30	
7:00	
7:30	
8:00	
8:30	
9:00	
9:30	
10:00	
10:30	
11:00	
11:30	
Noon	
12:30 p.m.	
1:00	
1:30	
2:00	
2:30	
3:00	
3:30	
4:00	
4:30	
5:00	
5:30	
6:00	
6:30	
7:00	
7:30	
8:00	
8:30	
9:00	
9:30	
10:00	
10:30	
11:00	

day 14

Get Ready for Tomorrow

date: _____

Today is your last day of preparation on the Beck Diet Solution program. Tomorrow, you will start your primary diet. To make sure you're ready, today you need to do the following tasks:

☐ Reread page 23 to remind yourself that you can modify your diet in advance to have small portions of whatever you want from time to time. So don't be tempted to overdo it today.

☐ Think of activities you'll need to do tomorrow and for the rest of the week. Will you have to go to the grocery store? Will you need extra time to prepare food? Will you pack a lunch and/or snacks?

☐ Prepare yourself psychologically for getting on the scale tomorrow. Think about the following: The number the scale registers isn't as important as the fact that you are now learning how to diet. Plan to weigh yourself first thing in the morning every day from now on.

☐ Look at the Sample (Partial) Food Plan Chart on page 80. You'll see that this dieter planned to have fruit and an omelet for breakfast: one medium apple (80 calories), 3 egg whites (52 calories) with 1 ounce Cheddar cheese (114 calories), and ¼ cup each of chopped pepper (8 calories) and chopped tomato (8 calories). Note that she didn't write down anything with 0 calories, such as her plain cup of tea and the nonstick spray she used to cook her omelet.

☐ Pull out the diet plan you chose last week, decide what you're going to eat tomorrow, and write everything on My Daily Food Plan Chart on page 83. Be sure to write in the precise amounts for each food and the number of units (calories, carbs, assigned points) if you're following a counting program. Cross off any snacks you don't plan to have.

☐ If you're tempted to skip this task, read Response Card #1 ("Do It Anyway").

Sample (Partial) Food Plan Chart

units allowed: <u>1,500</u> (calories)/carbs/assigned points

	Planned Eating Fill In Day Before and Check Off Immediately After Eating				Unplanned Eating Add Immediately After Eating		
	List Food	Amount	Units (calories, carbs, assigned points)	☑	List Food	Amount	Units (calories, carbs, assigned points)
breakfast	medium apple	1	80 cal				
	egg whites	3	52 cal				
	Cheddar cheese	1 ounce	114 cal				
	green pepper	¼ cup	8 cal				
	chopped tomato	¼ cup	8 cal				

what are you thinking?

Sabotaging Thought: I don't feel like planning and measuring my food. I know what and how much I'm going to eat. I don't need to go to so much effort.

Helpful Response: If I do only the things I feel like doing, I won't be able to lose weight and keep it off. Even if I don't need to do these things to lose weight initially, I have to learn how to make myself implement these crucial skills for the future, when my motivation to stick to my diet isn't as high as it is today.

today's to-do list

Each night, remember to check off each task you've completed. Circle any you didn't do, so you can be aware that you didn't follow the program completely.

☐ I read my list of reasons to lose weight (and other Response Cards as needed).

☐ I scheduled exercise and dieting activities on My Daily Schedule.

☐ I ate everything slowly and mindfully while sitting down.

☐ I exercised (for at least 5 to 30 minutes).

☐ I used distraction activities when I was hungry or having a craving.

☐ I filled out My Daily Food Plan Chart (page 83) for tomorrow's meals.

☐ I gave myself credit for these things and for: _____

_____

_____

_____

_____

_____.

My Daily Schedule

Use this chart to plan your diet and exercise activities for today.

Time	Activity
6:00 a.m.	
6:30	
7:00	
7:30	
8:00	
8:30	
9:00	
9:30	
10:00	
10:30	
11:00	
11:30	
Noon	
12:30 p.m.	
1:00	
1:30	
2:00	
2:30	
3:00	
3:30	
4:00	
4:30	
5:00	
5:30	
6:00	
6:30	
7:00	
7:30	
8:00	
8:30	
9:00	
9:30	
10:00	
10:30	
11:00	

My Daily Food Plan Chart

units allowed: _____ calories/carbs/assigned points

	Planned Eating Fill In Day Before and Check Off Immediately After Eating				**Unplanned Eating** Add Immediately After Eating		
	List Food	**Amount**	**Units** (calories, carbs, assigned points)	☑	**List Food**	**Amount**	**Units** (calories, carbs, assigned points)
breakfast							
snack							
lunch							
snack							
dinner							
snack							

units consumed: _____ calories/carbs/assigned points

chapter 7

Week 3

Let the Diet Begin!

You're ready to start your diet! How are you feeling? Excited? Apprehensive? Even if you've been dieting on and off for your whole life, this time will be different—if you learn and use the Beck Diet Solution skills. You'll practice one new Cognitive Therapy skill every day for the next month. I've already taught you some of them. Just think, when you dieted before, did you:

- Continually remind yourself of all of the reasons you have to lose weight?

- Respond effectively to your sabotaging thoughts?

- Choose a healthy diet plan and make reasonable modifications so you could stick to it?

- Use specific techniques to tolerate hunger, desires, and cravings?

- Consistently give yourself credit?

- Make enough time in your schedule to keep up with exercise?

In the past, you may have thought you'd lose weight if you just selected the right diet. But it's not the plan itself (as long as it's healthy and nutritious); *it's your ability to stick to it* that determines success. A study reported in *The Journal of the American Medical Association* (January 5, 2005) found that sticking to a diet is more important than the diet itself. I'll teach you "stick-to-it-iveness" so you can transform from someone who has struggled with dieting to a person who automatically does what he/she needs to do to achieve permanent weight loss.

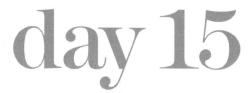

Start Your Diet

Today is a very important day—it's the first day of your diet! First, you need to establish a baseline weight. But before you get on the scale this morning, be sure to do the following:

☐ Tell yourself, *What the scale says today is not all that relevant because today is the first day of the rest of my new eating life ... In the future, my weight will go down because I'm finally* learning *how to diet.* Be careful not to criticize yourself. Remember that up to this point, you haven't had the skills to be successful in losing weight and/or maintaining weight loss. The important thing is *what you do from here on.*

☐ Weigh yourself before breakfast. Either wear no clothes or plan to wear the same weight of clothing when you weigh yourself every day in the future.

☐ Write down your weight here _____ or elsewhere. Even though you'll be weighing yourself daily, you'll record your change in weight just once a week, starting on Day 22 (see the graph on page 127).

☐ Follow the food plan you created yesterday (page 83), making sure you measure everything.

☐ When you finish eating, immediately check off what you ate on the food plan. Use the Sample (Partial) Food Plan Chart on page 86 as a guide.

☐ Give yourself credit for eating precisely what you had planned.

☐ If you eat something you hadn't planned or you eat a larger portion than you had planned, write it down in the unplanned section.

☐ Cross off any food you had planned to eat but didn't.

☐ Read the following Response Cards as often as needed to stay on track: #11 ("No Excuses"), #12 ("Resistance Habit"), #13 ("Can't Have It Both Ways"), #14 ("It's Not Okay"), #15 ("I'll Care Later"), and #16 ("I'd Rather Be Thinner"). Carry them around with you for the next month so you can read them whenever you're tempted to stray from your plan.

Check out how the dieter I worked with completed the breakfast part of her food plan. You'll see that she checked off the apple and most of the ingredients of her omelet. She crossed out the chopped tomato (because she didn't have any in the house) and wrote in ¼ cup chopped onion that she had on hand instead.

Sample (Partial) Food Plan Chart

units allowed: _1,500_ (calories)/carbs/assigned points

		Planned Eating Fill In Day Before and Check Off Immediately After Eating				Unplanned Eating Add Immediately After Eating		
	List Food	Amount	Units (calories, carbs, assigned points)	☑		List Food	Amount	Units (calories, carbs, assigned points)
breakfast	medium apple	1	80 cal	✓				
	egg whites	3	52 cal	✓				
	Cheddar cheese	1 ounce	114 cal	✓				
	green pepper	¼ cup	8 cal	✓				
	~~chopped tomato~~	~~¼ cup~~	~~8 cal~~			chopped onion	¼ cup	17 cal

Today, I'd also like you to start to journal about your eating experiences, to reinforce your good habits and to learn from your mistakes. (See the fill-in journaling space on page 88.) Plan to take just a couple of minutes a day to do this; it doesn't have to be extensive.

Here's how this dieter filled out her journal:

sample journal:

What did I do today to avoid unplanned eating? I brought my lunch to work.

 I reminded myself not to nibble as I was making dinner.

 I busied myself by e-mailing after dinner when I wanted to keep eating.

If I deviated, what happened? What can I learn from this for next time? I ate a free sample of

 food at the food market without thinking much about it. Next time, I'll remind

 myself before I even go into the store not to give in to unplanned eating.

Reflections: Today was easier than I expected. I can see how filling out the chart keeps

 me honest. I would have eaten Greg's pretzels this afternoon if I didn't have to

 write it down. I was momentarily disappointed that I couldn't eat the pretzels, but

 a few minutes later I felt GREAT that I had resisted. I really would SO much rather

 get thinner even though it means being disappointed now and then.

what are you thinking?

Sabotaging Thought: It's too much trouble to use the food plan chart. I don't really need it.

Helpful Response: I may not need it today, but I definitely will need it in the future. If I don't start learning this skill right now, chances are excellent that I'll regain whatever weight I lose.

today's to-do list

Each night, remember to check off each task you've completed. Circle any you didn't do, so you can be aware that you didn't follow the program completely.

☐ I weighed myself.

☐ I read my list of reasons to lose weight (and other Response Cards as needed).

☐ I scheduled exercise and dieting activities on My Daily Schedule.

☐ I measured all of my food.

☐ I ate everything slowly and mindfully while sitting down.

☐ I filled in my food plan *immediately* after eating.

☐ I stayed within my allotted units (calories, carbs, assigned points).

☐ I exercised (for at least 5 to 30 minutes).

☐ I used distraction techniques when I was hungry or having a craving.

☐ I contacted my diet coach today to say that I had started my diet.

☐ I filled in My Daily Food Plan Chart (page 90) for tomorrow's meals.

☐ I gave myself credit for these things and for: _____

_____

_____

_____

_____

_____ .

journal:

What did I do today to avoid unplanned eating? _____

_____

_____

_____

If I deviated, what happened? What can I learn from this for next time?_____

_____

_____

_____

Reflections: _____

_____

_____

_____

_____

_____

My Daily Schedule

Use this chart to plan your diet and exercise activities for today.

Time	Activity
6:00 a.m.	
6:30	
7:00	
7:30	
8:00	
8:30	
9:00	
9:30	
10:00	
10:30	
11:00	
11:30	
Noon	
12:30 p.m.	
1:00	
1:30	
2:00	
2:30	
3:00	
3:30	
4:00	
4:30	
5:00	
5:30	
6:00	
6:30	
7:00	
7:30	
8:00	
8:30	
9:00	
9:30	
10:00	
10:30	
11:00	

My Daily Food Plan Chart

units allowed: _____ calories/carbs/assigned points

		Planned Eating Fill In Day Before and Check Off Immediately After Eating				Unplanned Eating Add Immediately After Eating		
		List Food	Amount	Units (calories, carbs, assigned points)	☑	List Food	Amount	Units (calories, carbs, assigned points)
breakfast								
snack								
lunch								
snack								
dinner								
snack								

units consumed: _____ calories/carbs/assigned points

day 16

Say NO CHOICE to Unplanned Eating

One of the biggest challenges for dieters is to avoid unplanned eating—whether it's a desire to grab something out of the fridge or pantry while you're at home or a temptation to eat readily available food when you're out of the house. You have to recognize that you have to make a choice: You can eat what you want, when you want, *or* you can lose weight and keep it off—BUT YOU CAN'T DO BOTH.

☐ Put the issue of not giving in to eating unplanned foods in the NO CHOICE category, just as you have other must-do activities (for example, washing your face, brushing your teeth, combing your hair, and bathing). It doesn't matter if you feel like doing these things or not. You just don't give yourself a choice about them. You don't struggle. You just do them. Once you mentally commit to saying NO CHOICE to unplanned eating, you'll find that dieting is much easier. Carry around Response Card #17 ("NO CHOICE") for the next four weeks. Read it when you wake up and then throughout the day whenever you feel like eating something you haven't planned.

what are you thinking?

Sabotaging Thought: I want to be able to eat spontaneously sometimes.

Helpful Response: Then I have to accept the fact that I won't be able to keep off whatever weight I lose. The price of becoming and staying thinner is to follow whatever plan I establish for myself.

today's to-do list

Each night, remember to check off each task you've completed. Circle any you didn't do, so you can be aware that you didn't follow the program completely.

☐ I weighed myself.

☐ I read my list of reasons to lose weight (and other Response Cards as needed).

☐ I scheduled exercise and dieting activities on My Daily Schedule.

☐ I measured all of my food.

☐ I ate everything slowly and mindfully while sitting down.

☐ I filled in my food plan *immediately* after eating.

☐ I said NO CHOICE to food that I wasn't supposed to eat.

☐ I stayed within my allotted units (calories, carbs, assigned points).

☐ I exercised (for at least 5 to 30 minutes).

☐ I used distraction techniques when I was hungry or having a craving.

☐ I contacted my diet coach if I needed help.

☐ I filled in My Daily Food Plan Chart (page 95) for tomorrow's meals.

☐ I gave myself credit for these things and for: _____

_____

_____

_____

_____

_____ .

journal:

What did I do today to avoid unplanned eating? _____

_____

_____

_____

If I deviated, what happened? What can I learn from this for next time? _____

_____

_____

_____

Reflections: _____

_____

_____

_____

_____

_____

My Daily Schedule

Use this chart to plan your diet and exercise activities for today.

Time	Activity
6:00 a.m.	
6:30	
7:00	
7:30	
8:00	
8:30	
9:00	
9:30	
10:00	
10:30	
11:00	
11:30	
Noon	
12:30 p.m.	
1:00	
1:30	
2:00	
2:30	
3:00	
3:30	
4:00	
4:30	
5:00	
5:30	
6:00	
6:30	
7:00	
7:30	
8:00	
8:30	
9:00	
9:30	
10:00	
10:30	
11:00	

My Daily Food Plan Chart

units allowed: _____ calories/carbs/assigned points

	Planned Eating Fill In Day Before and Check Off Immediately After Eating				**Unplanned Eating** Add Immediately After Eating		
	List Food	**Amount**	**Units** (calories, carbs, assigned points)	☑	**List Food**	**Amount**	**Units** (calories, carbs, assigned points)
breakfast							
snack							
lunch							
snack							
dinner							
snack							

units consumed: _____ calories/carbs/assigned points

day 17

Learn to Stop Overeating

When you're not dieting, when do you usually stop eating? Is it when you finish all of the food on your plate? Is it after you have had seconds of whatever you want? Is it when the waistband on your clothes begins to feel tight?

Well, now you're going to need a different system. From now on, you're going to stop eating when the food you had planned to eat is gone (unless you planned to eat too much food to begin with). Since you won't always be able to control how much food you are served (such as when you eat out), I want you to practice wasting food. Do the following:

☐ Today, at breakfast and lunch, measure out your food carefully, as usual—but this time put extra portions on your plate.

☐ Before you begin eating, push those extra portions to one side and eat only what you had planned.

☐ If you're tempted to dig into the extra food, practice your distraction techniques from the chart on pages 76–77.

☐ When you finish the amount of food you were supposed to eat, stop eating and throw away the extras. Resist the temptation to just wrap them up. I want you to learn how to throw away food.

☐ Give yourself credit for not eating the extra food.

I'd also like you to prove to yourself that you shouldn't expect to feel full at the end of meals. It can take up to 20 minutes for a feeling of fullness to register. So do the following:

☐ Deliberately eat dinner very quickly today—and then stop.

☐ Immediately set a timer for 20 minutes.

☐ Read Response Card #10 ("If I'm Hungry After a Meal").

☐ Check off what you ate on your food plan as usual. Then get involved in other activities; you can choose some from My Distraction Techniques Chart if you want.

☐ When the timer goes off, assess your level of fullness. Is it different from when you first stopped eating?

It's very important for you to demonstrate to yourself the biological fact that satiety always kicks in—but that it does take time. If you don't learn this skill, then you're at risk for continuing to eat when your planned food is gone. If needed, repeat this task in the future.

what are you thinking?

Sabotaging Thought: I can't waste food.

Helpful Response: Then I'll always be in danger of gaining back whatever weight I lose. Throwing away food I'm not supposed to eat is an important skill. And I'll either waste food in the trash or waste it in my body as fat. Either way it's wasted.

today's to-do list

Each night, remember to check off each task you've completed. Circle any you didn't do, so you can be aware that you didn't follow the program completely.

☐ I weighed myself.

☐ I read my list of reasons to lose weight (and other Response Cards as needed).

☐ I scheduled exercise and dieting activities on My Daily Schedule.

☐ I measured all of my food.

☐ I ate everything slowly and mindfully while sitting down (except dinner).

☐ I filled in my food plan *immediately* after eating.

☐ I said NO CHOICE to food that I wasn't supposed to eat.

☐ I stayed within my allotted units (calories, carbs, assigned points).

☐ I exercised (for at least 5 to 30 minutes).

☐ I used distraction techniques when I was hungry or having a craving.

☐ I contacted my diet coach if I needed help.

☐ I refrained from overeating.

☐ I practiced throwing away food.

☐ I filled in My Daily Food Plan Chart (page 100) for tomorrow's meals.

☐ I gave myself credit for these things and for: _____

_____

_____

_____

_____

_____ .

journal:

What did I do today to avoid unplanned eating? _____

_____

_____

_____

If I deviated, what happened? What can I learn from this for next time?_____

_____

_____

_____

Reflections: _____

_____

_____

_____

_____

My Daily Schedule

Use this chart to plan your diet and exercise activities for today.

Time	Activity
6:00 a.m.	
6:30	
7:00	
7:30	
8:00	
8:30	
9:00	
9:30	
10:00	
10:30	
11:00	
11:30	
Noon	
12:30 p.m.	
1:00	
1:30	
2:00	
2:30	
3:00	
3:30	
4:00	
4:30	
5:00	
5:30	
6:00	
6:30	
7:00	
7:30	
8:00	
8:30	
9:00	
9:30	
10:00	
10:30	
11:00	

My Daily Food Plan Chart

units allowed: _____ calories/carbs/assigned points

| | | | Planned Eating | | Unplanned Eating | | |
| | | | Fill In Day Before and Check Off Immediately After Eating | | Add Immediately After Eating | | |

	List Food	Amount	Units (calories, carbs, assigned points)	☑	List Food	Amount	Units (calories, carbs, assigned points)
breakfast							
snack							
lunch							
snack							
dinner							
snack							

units consumed: _____ calories/carbs/assigned points

day 18

Redefine Full

M any chronic dieters need to change their concept of fullness because they continue to eat even *after* the sensation of fullness sets in. To learn how to avoid this problem, take these steps:

☐ Consistently spread in front of you all of the food you've planned to eat at a meal, all at once, before you start eating (as described on page 96). When you do so today, take a look. Have you planned to eat greater quantities of unlimited or low-calorie foods than you really need?

☐ If you suspect the answer is yes, you may be stocking up, worried that if you don't eat enough, you'll be too hungry before your next meal. If so, read Response Card #8 ("Tolerate It!") and do the dinner task on Day 17 (page 96) again.

☐ After you finish each meal today, ask yourself whether you'd be able to take a brisk walk. If the answer is no and you feel mildly bloated or lethargic, it may mean that you've actually eaten too much.

☐ If you feel disappointed that you can't eat more after finishing a meal, remind yourself that it's okay—you'll be able to have a meal (or a snack, if you planned one) in just a few hours. It's actually good to be hungry at times because it gives you a chance to build up your tolerance.

what are you thinking?

Sabotaging Thought: I really enjoy eating a lot of food. What's the harm in eating lots of low-calorie or "free" foods?

Helpful Response: There is potential harm. I have to get used to what normal fullness feels like. Although I may fill up on low-calorie foods today, at some point I'll be tempted to fill up on other foods. I really want to learn to be a normal eater.

today's to-do list

Each night, remember to check off each task you've completed. Circle any you didn't do, so you can be aware that you didn't follow the program completely.

☐ I weighed myself.

☐ I read my list of reasons to lose weight (and other Response Cards as needed).

☐ I scheduled exercise and dieting activities on My Daily Schedule.

☐ I measured all of my food.

☐ I ate everything slowly and mindfully while sitting down.

☐ I filled in my food plan *immediately* after eating.

☐ I said NO CHOICE to food that I wasn't supposed to eat.

☐ I stayed within my allotted units (calories, carbs, assigned points).

☐ I exercised (for at least 5 to 30 minutes).

☐ I used distraction techniques when I was hungry or having a craving.

☐ I contacted my diet coach if I needed help.

☐ I refrained from overeating.

☐ I filled in My Daily Food Plan Chart (page 105) for tomorrow's meals.

☐ I gave myself credit for these things and for: _____

_____

_____

_____

_____

_____ .

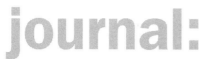 journal:

What did I do today to avoid unplanned eating? _____

_____

_____

_____

If I deviated, what happened? What can I learn from this for next time? _____

_____

_____

_____

Reflections: _____

_____

_____

_____

_____

My Daily Schedule

Use this chart to plan your diet and exercise activities for today.

Time	Activity
6:00 a.m.	
6:30	
7:00	
7:30	
8:00	
8:30	
9:00	
9:30	
10:00	
10:30	
11:00	
11:30	
Noon	
12:30 p.m.	
1:00	
1:30	
2:00	
2:30	
3:00	
3:30	
4:00	
4:30	
5:00	
5:30	
6:00	
6:30	
7:00	
7:30	
8:00	
8:30	
9:00	
9:30	
10:00	
10:30	
11:00	

My Daily Food Plan Chart

units allowed: _____ calories/carbs/assigned points

	Planned Eating Fill In Day Before and Check Off Immediately After Eating				**Unplanned Eating** Add Immediately After Eating		
	List Food	Amount	Units (calories, carbs, assigned points)	☑	List Food	Amount	Units (calories, carbs, assigned points)
breakfast							
snack							
lunch							
snack							
dinner							
snack							

units consumed: _____ calories/carbs/assigned points

date: _____

day 19

Don't Deceive Yourself

U nsuccessful dieters have usually perfected a particular skill: the ability to delude themselves about their eating. You may be completely logical and rational about other areas of your life. But when it comes to food, you try to justify every unplanned bite you take. Do the following:

☐ As you go through the day today, see if you have a desire to eat something that's not on your plan and pay special attention to any thoughts you have that start with, *It's okay to eat this because....*

☐ Read Response Cards #11 ("No Excuses"), #12 ("Resistance Habit"), #13 ("Can't Have It Both Ways"), #14 ("It's Not Okay"), #15 ("I'll Care Later"), #16 ("I'd Rather Be Thinner"), and #17 ("NO CHOICE") whenever you find yourself trying to justify eating unplanned food.

Another way dieters deceive themselves is by underestimating how much they're eating. First, they sometimes fool themselves by not counting all of the ingredients in their food. Second, they eyeball their food instead of measuring it.

Before you serve yourself any food today, do the following:

☐ Look closely at all of the food in your meals and snacks. Are you sure that you've written down *every* ingredient in every dish? For example, did you remember to write down the oil, butter, or mayonnaise used in the preparation of such foods as scrambled eggs, tuna or chicken salad, or sautéed vegetables?

☐ Don't premeasure your meals and snacks today. Get your food ready and then write down what you *think* it weighs (or, if applicable, how many teaspoons or cups it is) on My Food Chart on the facing page. Use the Sample Food Chart one dieter filled out above it as an example.

☐ Next, get out your kitchen scale and measuring spoons and cups. Measure all of your foods and write down the actual measurements on your chart. See how close you actually were.

Sample Food Chart

Food	Estimated Measurement	Actual Measurement
cottage cheese	½ cup	¾ cup
grapes	1 cup	1½ cups
tuna	3 ounces	4 ounces
mayonnaise	1 teaspoon	1 teaspoon
chicken breast	5 ounces	6 ounces
green beans	1½ cups	1¼ cups
rice	½ cup	¾ cup
popcorn	2 cups	3 cups

My Food Chart

Food	Estimated Measurement	Actual Measurement

what are you thinking?

Sabotaging Thought: It's okay to eat this food that I haven't planned to eat because....

Helpful Response: I have to become an expert at resisting all foods that I haven't planned to eat. If I want to lose weight and keep it off, I just can't eat what I want unless it's on my plan.

today's to-do list

Each night, remember to check off each task you've completed. Circle any you didn't do, so you can be aware that you didn't follow the program completely.

☐ I weighed myself.

☐ I read my list of reasons to lose weight (and other Response Cards as needed).

☐ I scheduled exercise and dieting activities on My Daily Schedule.

☐ I measured all of my food.

☐ I ate everything slowly and mindfully while sitting down.

☐ I refrained from overeating.

☐ I filled in my food plan *immediately* after eating.

☐ I said NO CHOICE to food that I wasn't supposed to eat.

☐ I stayed within my allotted units (calories, carbs, assigned points).

☐ I exercised (for at least 5 to 30 minutes).

☐ I used distraction techniques when I was hungry or having a craving.

☐ I contacted my diet coach if I needed help.

☐ I was alert for "fooling myself" thoughts.

☐ I filled in My Daily Food Plan Chart (page 111) for tomorrow's meals.

☐ I gave myself credit for these things and for: _____

_____

_____

_____

_____

_____.

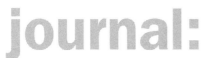

journal:

What did I do today to avoid unplanned eating? _____

_____

_____

_____

If I deviated, what happened? What can I learn from this for next time?_____

_____

_____

_____

Reflections: _____

_____

_____

_____

_____

_____

My Daily Schedule

Use this chart to plan your diet and exercise activities for today.

Time	Activity
6:00 a.m.	
6:30	
7:00	
7:30	
8:00	
8:30	
9:00	
9:30	
10:00	
10:30	
11:00	
11:30	
Noon	
12:30 p.m.	
1:00	
1:30	
2:00	
2:30	
3:00	
3:30	
4:00	
4:30	
5:00	
5:30	
6:00	
6:30	
7:00	
7:30	
8:00	
8:30	
9:00	
9:30	
10:00	
10:30	
11:00	

My Daily Food Plan Chart

units allowed: _____ calories/carbs/assigned points

	Planned Eating Fill In Day Before and Check Off Immediately After Eating				**Unplanned Eating** Add Immediately After Eating		
	List Food	**Amount**	**Units** (calories, carbs, assigned points)	☑	**List Food**	**Amount**	**Units** (calories, carbs, assigned points)
breakfast							
snack							
lunch							
snack							
dinner							
snack							

units consumed: _____ calories/carbs/assigned points

day 20

Start Over This Moment

One particular kind of thinking can really create havoc on your diet—the thought you have when you have eaten something unplanned: *I might as well abandon my diet and eat whatever I want for the rest of the day.* To get ready to battle this idea, think about the following: Is it better to stop eating when you've made a 200- to 300-calorie mistake or when you've made a 2,000- to 3,000-calorie mistake? Since you can choose to stop at any point, why not stop as soon as possible? Why compound one mistake with another? Mark this page so that you can turn to it immediately when you make your first eating mistake. Here's what you'll need to do:

- ☐ Tell yourself, *Okay, I shouldn't have eaten that, but I'm not going to let this one mistake ruin my diet.*

- ☐ Recommit to your diet then and there: *I am going to go back to my plan, right now, for the rest of the day ... It makes no sense to wait till tomorrow ... If I do, I'll just gain weight.*

- ☐ Draw a line, symbolically, by changing gears and immediately engaging in several of your distraction activities (pages 76–77) to get your mind off your mistake and to prevent further unplanned eating.

- ☐ Give yourself credit for stopping at any point. Congratulations—it's a significant accomplishment to get right back on your eating plan after you've strayed from it!

- ☐ Read Response Card #18 ("Get Back on Track") as often as needed.

- ☐ Take a 20- to 30-minute walk. You will feel so much better about yourself psychologically—and your food will metabolize faster.

what are you thinking?

Sabotaging Thought: How could I have eaten that? I'm never going to succeed at dieting. I should just give up now.

Helpful Response: I'm not going to let this minor setback ruin everything I've accomplished. One mistake does not ruin my diet, but falling back into old patterns *will.* I'm recommitting to my diet right here, right now.

today's to-do list

Each night, remember to check off each task you've completed. Circle any you didn't do, so you can be aware that you didn't follow the program completely.

☐ I weighed myself.

☐ I read my list of reasons to lose weight (and other Response Cards as needed).

☐ I scheduled exercise and dieting activities on My Daily Schedule.

☐ I measured all of my food.

☐ I ate everything slowly and mindfully while sitting down.

☐ I refrained from overeating.

☐ I filled in my food plan *immediately* after eating.

☐ I said NO CHOICE to food that I wasn't supposed to eat.

☐ I stayed within my allotted units (calories, carbs, assigned points).

☐ I exercised (for at least 5 to 30 minutes).

☐ I used distraction techniques when I was hungry or having a craving.

☐ I contacted my diet coach if I needed help.

☐ I was alert for "fooling myself" thoughts.

☐ I prepared myself to get back on track when I make eating mistakes.

☐ I filled in My Daily Food Plan Chart (page 116) for tomorrow's meals.

☐ I gave myself credit for these things and for: _____

_____

_____

_____

_____

_____ .

journal:

What did I do today to avoid unplanned eating? _____

_____

_____

_____

If I deviated, what happened? What can I learn from this for next time? _____

_____

_____

_____

Reflections: _____

_____

_____

_____

_____

_____

My Daily Schedule

Use this chart to plan your diet and exercise activities for today.

Time	Activity
6:00 a.m.	
6:30	
7:00	
7:30	
8:00	
8:30	
9:00	
9:30	
10:00	
10:30	
11:00	
11:30	
Noon	
12:30 p.m.	
1:00	
1:30	
2:00	
2:30	
3:00	
3:30	
4:00	
4:30	
5:00	
5:30	
6:00	
6:30	
7:00	
7:30	
8:00	
8:30	
9:00	
9:30	
10:00	
10:30	
11:00	

My Daily Food Plan Chart

units allowed: _____ calories/carbs/assigned points

	Planned Eating — Fill In Day Before and Check Off Immediately After Eating				Unplanned Eating — Add Immediately After Eating		
	List Food	Amount	Units (calories, carbs, assigned points)	☑	List Food	Amount	Units (calories, carbs, assigned points)
breakfast							
snack							
lunch							
snack							
dinner							
snack							

units consumed: _____ calories/carbs/assigned points

day 21

Prepare for the Scale

When you weigh yourself tomorrow, you're going to mark the amount you lost on your weight-loss graph (page 127). You'll continue to graph your change in weight at the end of each week, Now, do the following:

☐ Put a sticky note on page 127 so that you can find it easily in the future.

☐ Note the dot at 0. Tomorrow morning, you'll calculate the difference in your weight since last week and mark it on the graph above "Week 1." Then you'll draw a line from the original dot to the new dot. Continue to weigh yourself every day to stay in touch with your progress but record your change in weight only once a week.

☐ Today, get yourself ready psychologically. Remember, you should aim for a ½- to 2-pound weight loss most weeks. Anything in that range is considered normal and is an achievement that should make you proud. Read Response Card #19 ("Celebrate!").

what are you thinking?

Sabotaging Thought: I should lose a lot of weight very quickly.

Helpful Response: Losing weight too quickly may mean my diet isn't healthy enough. If I keep my expectations realistic, I'll feel good when I get on the scale. If I'm unrealistic, I'll feel bad and be more likely to give up.

today's to-do list

Each night, remember to check off each task you've completed. Circle any you didn't do, so you can be aware that you didn't follow the program completely.

☐ I weighed myself.

☐ I read my list of reasons to lose weight (and other Response Cards as needed).

☐ I scheduled exercise and dieting activities on My Daily Schedule.

☐ I measured all of my food.

☐ I ate everything slowly and mindfully while sitting down.

☐ I refrained from overeating.

☐ I filled in my food plan *immediately* after eating.

☐ I said NO CHOICE to food that I wasn't supposed to eat.

☐ I stayed within my allotted units (calories, carbs, assigned points).

☐ I exercised (for at least 5 to 30 minutes).

☐ I used distraction techniques when I was hungry or having a craving.

☐ I contacted my diet coach if I needed help.

☐ I was alert for "fooling myself" thoughts.

☐ I prepared myself to get back on track when I make eating mistakes.

☐ I filled in My Daily Food Plan Chart (page 121) for tomorrow's meals.

☐ I gave myself credit for these things and for: _____

_____

_____

_____

_____

_____.

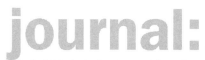

journal:

What did I do today to avoid unplanned eating? _____

_____

_____

_____

If I deviated, what happened? What can I learn from this for next time?_____

_____

_____

_____

Reflections: _____

_____

_____

_____

_____

My Daily Schedule

Use this chart to plan your diet and exercise activities for today.

Time	Activity
6:00 a.m.	
6:30	
7:00	
7:30	
8:00	
8:30	
9:00	
9:30	
10:00	
10:30	
11:00	
11:30	
Noon	
12:30 p.m.	
1:00	
1:30	
2:00	
2:30	
3:00	
3:30	
4:00	
4:30	
5:00	
5:30	
6:00	
6:30	
7:00	
7:30	
8:00	
8:30	
9:00	
9:30	
10:00	
10:30	
11:00	

My Daily Food Plan Chart

units allowed: _____ calories/carbs/assigned points

	Planned Eating Fill In Day Before and Check Off Immediately After Eating				**Unplanned Eating** Add Immediately After Eating		
	List Food	**Amount**	**Units** (calories, carbs, assigned points)	☑	**List Food**	**Amount**	**Units** (calories, carbs, assigned points)
breakfast							
snack							
lunch							
snack							
dinner							
snack							

units consumed: _____ calories/carbs/assigned points

chapter 8

Week 4

Fight Undermining Ideas

I hope you feel proud of yourself and are giving yourself credit for the way you've incorporated new skills from the Beck Diet Solution to stay on track. You *should* be proud—that's a major accomplishment. Now, it's time to anticipate and plan for the harder times, when you will inevitably feel a sense of unfairness, deprivation, disappointment, or discouragement. These are the times when you may be sorely tempted to stop following your plan, but developing specific skills to deal with these issues will enable you to get through the tough times unscathed. You'll end up being so pleased with yourself that you were able to continue losing weight instead of gaining it back.

day 22

Learn the Power of *Oh, Well*

Today is the day to record your change in weight on My Weight-Loss Graph on page 127. Remember to wear the same weight of clothing you wore when you weighed yourself on Day 15.

☐ Weigh yourself before breakfast and draw a line on the graph showing how much you lost or gained this week.

☐ Call your diet coach and report your change in weight. If you haven't lost weight, ask for help in solving the problem. It may mean you need to cut your calories or to increase your exercise. Make sure you've been counting every bite of food you eat.

☐ If you have lost weight, read Response Card #19 ("Celebrate!").

☐ If you're disappointed with your weight loss, practice the *Oh, well* technique below.

Almost every dieter becomes disappointed at some point. When you started this diet a week ago, you may have been full of enthusiasm and willing to do whatever it takes to lose weight. I hope you still feel that way. But I can predict that at some point you will feel disappointed, especially if you really want to eat something you haven't planned, if you feel like skipping exercise, or if your weight loss isn't progressing as quickly as you'd like.

I'd like you to start practicing a skill now to deal with disappointment so that later you don't end up overeating and perhaps abandoning your diet. Here's what I want you to do:

☐ When you start to feel deprived or disgruntled about having to restrict your food, work toward acceptance: *If I want to lose weight/be thinner/be healthier/feel better about myself/have more energy/fit into clothes better/have more self-confidence/be less self-conscious/be proud of myself then I have to accept the fact that the only way I can achieve these benefits is to restrict my eating. I just can't have it both ways. That's just not possible.*

☐ Say *Oh, well*, which means, *I don't like this, but I can't change it, so I'll accept it and move on.*

☐ Try to identify whether you already say the equivalent of *Oh, well* to yourself when you do something you don't want to do, such as getting out of bed in the morning, paying your bills, or cleaning the house. If these are activities you don't enjoy, you often just accept the necessity of doing them. That's what I want you to do with the disappointment you will occasionally feel about dieting.

☐ Carry Response Card #20 ("Oh, Well") with you to remind yourself to use this technique whenever you need it.

what are you thinking?

Sabotaging Thought: I don't want to accept the restrictions. There must be an easier way.

Helpful Response: Nonacceptance is going to lead to struggle, and I'll probably give up and regain any weight I lose. I have to accept the fact that there is no easier way.

today's to-do list

Each night, remember to check off each task you've completed. Circle any you didn't do, so you can be aware that you didn't follow the program completely.

☐ I weighed myself and reported the change in my weight to my coach.

☐ I read my list of reasons to lose weight (and other Response Cards as needed).

☐ I scheduled exercise and dieting activities on My Daily Schedule.

☐ I measured all of my food.

☐ I ate everything slowly and mindfully while sitting down.

☐ I refrained from overeating.

☐ I filled in my food plan *immediately* after eating.

☐ I said NO CHOICE to food that I wasn't supposed to eat.

☐ I stayed within my allotted units (calories, carbs, assigned points).

☐ I exercised (for at least 5 to 30 minutes).

☐ I used distraction techniques when I was hungry or having a craving.

☐ I contacted my diet coach if I needed help.

☐ I was alert for "fooling myself" thoughts.

☐ I used the *Oh, well* technique to deal with disappointment (if needed).

☐ I filled in My Daily Food Plan Chart (page 129) for tomorrow's meals.

☐ I gave myself credit for these things and for: _____

_____

_____

_____

_____

_____.

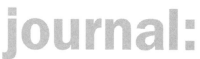

journal:

What did I do today to avoid unplanned eating? _____

_____

_____

_____

If I deviated, what happened? What can I learn from this for next time? _____

_____

_____

_____

Reflections: _____

_____

_____

_____

_____

_____

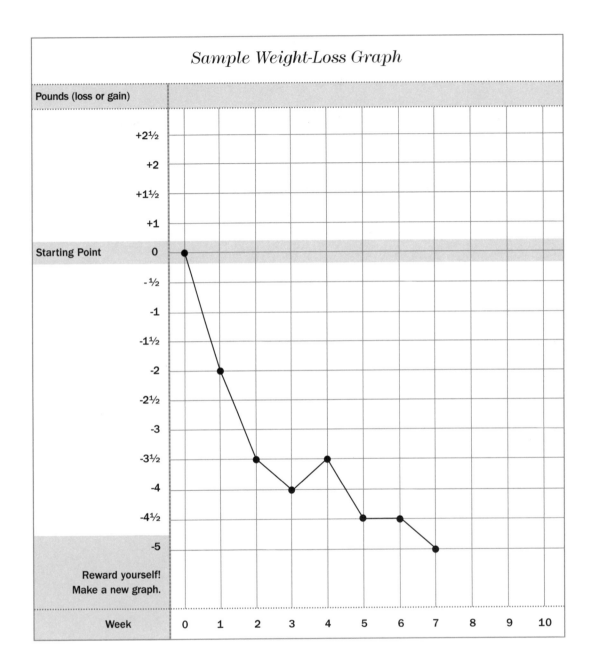

Sample Weight-Loss Graph

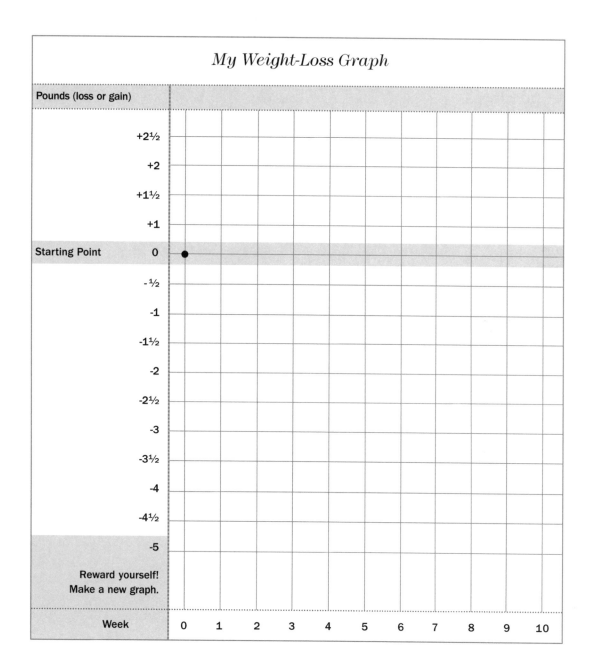

My Weight-Loss Graph

Pounds (loss or gain)

	+2½
	+2
	+1½
	+1
Starting Point	0
	-½
	-1
	-1½
	-2
	-2½
	-3
	-3½
	-4
	-4½
	-5

Reward yourself!
Make a new graph.

Week   0   1   2   3   4   5   6   7   8   9   10

My Daily Schedule

Use this chart to plan your diet and exercise activities for today.

Time	Activity
6:00 a.m.	
6:30	
7:00	
7:30	
8:00	
8:30	
9:00	
9:30	
10:00	
10:30	
11:00	
11:30	
Noon	
12:30 p.m.	
1:00	
1:30	
2:00	
2:30	
3:00	
3:30	
4:00	
4:30	
5:00	
5:30	
6:00	
6:30	
7:00	
7:30	
8:00	
8:30	
9:00	
9:30	
10:00	
10:30	
11:00	

My Daily Food Plan Chart

units allowed: _____ calories/carbs/assigned points

	Planned Eating Fill In Day Before and Check Off Immediately After Eating				Unplanned Eating Add Immediately After Eating		
	List Food	Amount	Units (calories, carbs, assigned points)	☑	List Food	Amount	Units (calories, carbs, assigned points)
breakfast							
snack							
lunch							
snack							
dinner							
snack							

units consumed: _____ calories/carbs/assigned points

day 23

Overcome Feelings of Unfairness

Life isn't fair, that's for sure. It seems even less fair when you have to restrict your eating. A lot of people get in trouble when they use the unfairness issue as an excuse to deviate from their diet: *It's not fair that I can't eat this food ... Life should be fair ... Therefore, I am going to eat it.*

Check off any thoughts below that you've had in the past or that you're likely to have in the future: It's unfair that:

- ☐ I have to deprive myself so much.
- ☐ I can't eat like other people.
- ☐ I have to work so hard to lose weight.
- ☐ I have such a lousy metabolism.
- ☐ A tendency toward being overweight runs in my family.
- ☐ I can't be spontaneous in my eating.
- ☐ I have to monitor what I eat.

All true: None of these things is fair. But you have two choices about how you can react to this unfairness. I'd like you to think hard about both of them:

1. You can feel sorry for yourself, stray from your diet, never end up losing weight, and continue to be unhappy.

2. Or you can sympathize with those feelings, accept what you have to do to lose weight, go ahead and do it, lose the weight, enjoy all of the benefits of that weight loss, feel strong and in control, and be proud of yourself.

Which do you choose? To make this issue a little easier, do these things:

- ☐ Read your list of reasons to lose weight and think about all of the wonderful benefits you'll get from sticking to your diet.

- ☐ Think about the following: Is it better to struggle about unfairness—or accept it and move on? After all, everyone has unfair parts of life. This is just one of yours. Besides, wouldn't the greatest unfairness be to allow the "unfairness excuse" to prevent you from losing weight?

☐ Put unfairness in perspective by making a mental note of the positive things in your life. Focus on the fact that doing something to improve your health is one of the most fair and reasonable things you can do for yourself.

what are you thinking?

Sabotaging Thought: Why does eating have to be unfair? I guess I understand it, but I really don't like having to live with it.

Helpful Response: That's okay. Of course I don't like it now. But I'll be very happy that I learned to accept unfairness when I've lost weight and been able to keep it off.

today's to-do list

Each night, remember to check off each task you've completed. Circle any you didn't do, so you can be aware that you didn't follow the program completely.

☐ I weighed myself.

☐ I read my list of reasons to lose weight (and other Response Cards as needed).

☐ I scheduled exercise and dieting activities on My Daily Schedule.

☐ I measured all of my food.

☐ I ate everything slowly and mindfully while sitting down.

☐ I refrained from overeating.

☐ I filled in my food plan *immediately* after eating.

☐ I said NO CHOICE to food that I wasn't supposed to eat.

☐ I stayed within my allotted units (calories, carbs, assigned points).

☐ I exercised (for at least 5 to 30 minutes).

☐ I used distraction techniques when I was hungry or having a craving.

☐ I contacted my diet coach if I needed help.

☐ I was alert for "fooling myself" thoughts.

☐ I used the *Oh, well* technique to deal with disappointment (if needed).

☐ I prepared myself for the "unfairness" issue.

☐ I filled in My Daily Food Plan Chart (page 134) for tomorrow's meals.

☐ I gave myself credit for these things and for: _____

_____

_____

_____

_____

_____.

journal:

What did I do today to avoid unplanned eating? _____

_____

_____

_____

If I deviated, what happened? What can I learn from this for next time? _____

_____

_____

_____

Reflections: _____

_____

_____

_____

_____

My Daily Schedule

Use this chart to plan your diet and exercise activities for today.

Time	Activity
6:00 a.m.	
6:30	
7:00	
7:30	
8:00	
8:30	
9:00	
9:30	
10:00	
10:30	
11:00	
11:30	
Noon	
12:30 p.m.	
1:00	
1:30	
2:00	
2:30	
3:00	
3:30	
4:00	
4:30	
5:00	
5:30	
6:00	
6:30	
7:00	
7:30	
8:00	
8:30	
9:00	
9:30	
10:00	
10:30	
11:00	

My Daily Food Plan Chart

units allowed: _____ calories/carbs/assigned points

	Planned Eating Fill In Day Before and Check Off Immediately After Eating				Unplanned Eating Add Immediately After Eating		
	List Food	Amount	Units (calories, carbs, assigned points)	☑	List Food	Amount	Units (calories, carbs, assigned points)
breakfast							
snack							
lunch							
snack							
dinner							
snack							

units consumed: _____ calories/carbs/assigned points

date: _____

Diminish Discouragement

It's normal to experience feelings of discouragement from time to time when you're dieting. At some point, you'll begin to think it's not worth all of the effort. This can happen when you:

- Struggle over restricting your eating or doing other diet-related tasks.

- Make a momentary slip by overeating or engaging in unplanned eating.

- Become overwhelmed at the prospect of using your dieting techniques and restricting your eating over the long term.

- Get on the scale and see that you haven't lost weight.

Don't let feelings of discouragement become an excuse for you to stray from your diet. Here's what you can do:

☐ Read your list of reasons to lose weight a little more often. Remember, the rewards of being thinner will be so much greater than the discomfort of continuing your efforts.

☐ At the end of the day, reflect on how much time you spent feeling discouraged. Most dieters I work with say that they actually only felt discouraged for 20 to 30 minutes at a time, and then the feeling passed. That's not a lot of time in the scheme of things. Remind yourself that discouragement is temporary.

☐ Don't think too much about the future. Dieting "forever" sounds extremely hard. Dieting "just for today" is doable.

☐ If you slip up, remind yourself that mistakes happen—nobody is perfect. The important thing is how you deal with your mistake. You can get discouraged and compound the mistake by eating more, or you can decide to get right back on track.

☐ Read Response Card #21 ("Advice to a Friend").

Remember that dieting is *supposed* to be hard at times. But keep in mind, too, that it will soon get so much easier—then you'll just have brief times when it's difficult again.

what are you thinking?

Sabotaging Thought: I'm just not sure I can do it. It's so much work.

Helpful Response: It *is* a lot of work, but it will get easier once the skills I'm learning get to be second nature. It's worth doing to get all the advantages of weight loss.

today's to-do list

Each night, remember to check off each task you've completed. Circle any you didn't do, so you can be aware that you didn't follow the program completely.

☐ I weighed myself.

☐ I read my list of reasons to lose weight (and other Response Cards as needed).

☐ I scheduled exercise and dieting activities on My Daily Schedule.

☐ I measured all of my food before I ate.

☐ I stayed within my allotted units (calories, carbs, assigned points).

☐ I ate everything slowly and mindfully while sitting down and refrained from overeating.

☐ I filled in my food plan *immediately* after eating.

☐ I said NO CHOICE to food that I wasn't supposed to eat.

☐ I exercised (for at least 5 to 30 minutes).

☐ I used distraction techniques when I was hungry or having a craving.

☐ I contacted my diet coach if I needed help.

☐ I used the *Oh, well* technique to deal with disappointment (if needed).

☐ I filled in My Daily Food Plan Chart (page 139) for tomorrow's meals.

☐ I gave myself credit for these things and for: _____

_____

_____

_____

_____

_____ .

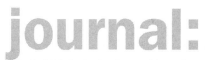

journal:

What did I do today to avoid unplanned eating? _____

_____

_____

_____

If I deviated, what happened? What can I learn from this for next time? _____

_____

_____

_____

Reflections: _____

_____

_____

_____

_____

My Daily Schedule

Use this chart to plan your diet and exercise activities for today.

Time	Activity
6:00 a.m.	
6:30	
7:00	
7:30	
8:00	
8:30	
9:00	
9:30	
10:00	
10:30	
11:00	
11:30	
Noon	
12:30 p.m.	
1:00	
1:30	
2:00	
2:30	
3:00	
3:30	
4:00	
4:30	
5:00	
5:30	
6:00	
6:30	
7:00	
7:30	
8:00	
8:30	
9:00	
9:30	
10:00	
10:30	
11:00	

My Daily Food Plan Chart

units allowed: _____ calories/carbs/assigned points

	Planned Eating Fill In Day Before and Check Off Immediately After Eating				Unplanned Eating Add Immediately After Eating		
	List Food	Amount	Units (calories, carbs, assigned points)	☑	List Food	Amount	Units (calories, carbs, assigned points)
breakfast							
snack							
lunch							
snack							
dinner							
snack							

units consumed: _____ calories/carbs/assigned points

day 25

Pay Attention to Your Thinking

Your thoughts are very powerful. You've already read many examples of how your thinking can lead you to stray from your diet. Left unaddressed, at some point sabotaging thoughts could lead you to abandon your diet altogether. Now, I'd like you to start identifying and tracking those sabotaging thoughts—and keep up this practice indefinitely.

Here's how you'll know if you're having a sabotaging thought:

- You feel tempted to eat something you shouldn't.

- You actually eat something you shouldn't.

- You feel tempted to skip doing some part of the Beck Diet Solution program.

- You feel unhappy about some element of dieting.

☐ At these times, ask yourself, *What was just going through my mind? What was I just thinking?*

☐ Record these thoughts in today's journaling section.

And, remember, you can stop yourself from unplanned eating and engaging in other diet-sabotaging behavior by talking back to your thoughts. You'll learn how to refine this skill in the next two days.

what are you thinking?

Sabotaging Thought: Most of the time I'm not thinking anything specific. I just feel down or discouraged.

Helpful Response: Actually I *am* having thoughts that are either leading me to feel this way or are making me feel worse. The more I practice, the better I'll get at figuring out my thinking.

today's to-do list

Each night, remember to check off each task you've completed. Circle any you didn't do, so you can be aware that you didn't follow the program completely.

☐ I weighed myself.

☐ I read my list of reasons to lose weight (and other Response Cards as needed).

☐ I scheduled exercise and dieting activities on My Daily Schedule.

☐ I measured all of my food before I ate.

☐ I stayed within my allotted units (calories, carbs, assigned points).

☐ I ate everything slowly and mindfully while sitting down and refrained from overeating.

☐ I filled in my food plan *immediately* after eating.

☐ I said NO CHOICE to food that I wasn't supposed to eat.

☐ I exercised (for at least 5 to 30 minutes).

☐ I used distraction techniques when I was hungry or having a craving.

☐ I contacted my diet coach if I needed help.

☐ I used the *Oh, well* technique to deal with disappointment (if needed).

☐ I filled in My Daily Food Plan Chart (page 144) for tomorrow's meals.

☐ I gave myself credit for these things and for: _____

_____

_____

_____

_____

_____.

journal:

What did I do today to avoid unplanned eating? _____

_____

_____

_____

If I deviated, what happened? _____

_____

_____

_____

What sabotaging thoughts did I have? _____

_____

_____

_____

What can I learn from this for next time? _____

_____

_____

_____

Reflections: _____

_____

_____

_____

_____

My Daily Schedule

Use this chart to plan your diet and exercise activities for today.

Time	Activity
6:00 a.m.	
6:30	
7:00	
7:30	
8:00	
8:30	
9:00	
9:30	
10:00	
10:30	
11:00	
11:30	
Noon	
12:30 p.m.	
1:00	
1:30	
2:00	
2:30	
3:00	
3:30	
4:00	
4:30	
5:00	
5:30	
6:00	
6:30	
7:00	
7:30	
8:00	
8:30	
9:00	
9:30	
10:00	
10:30	
11:00	

My Daily Food Plan Chart

units allowed: _____ calories/carbs/assigned points

	Planned Eating Fill In Day Before and Check Off Immediately After Eating				Unplanned Eating Add Immediately After Eating		
	List Food	Amount	Units (calories, carbs, assigned points)	☑	List Food	Amount	Units (calories, carbs, assigned points)
breakfast							
snack							
lunch							
snack							
dinner							
snack							

units consumed: _____ calories/carbs/assigned points

day 26

Identify and Correct Thinking Errors

Remember what we discussed in Chapter 1, that just because you think something does not necessarily mean it's true? For example, you may think, *My friends will be disappointed if I don't drink at the party*. Yet, in reality, some of them may not notice or care. Or your thoughts could be completely untrue: *I have to eat ... I can't stand being hungry*. Recognizing and correcting inaccurate thoughts is an essential skill to master if you want to keep losing weight and to maintain your weight loss.

People tend to make very predictable errors in their thinking. Typical errors of dieters appear in the chart on pages 146–147. Do the following:

☐ Read each item in the Thinking Mistakes Chart and make Response Cards for any you think will be useful.

☐ When recording sabotaging thoughts in today's journal section, see if you can identify particular thinking errors. Don't worry if you can't; it's a useful but not essential skill.

☐ Reference this chart often; it will help you create responses to your sabotaging thoughts.

Thinking Mistakes Chart

Thinking Mistakes	Description	Example	Helpful Response
All-or-nothing thinking	You see things in only two categories when it is really on a continuum.	*Either I'm perfect on my diet or I've completely failed.*	*Making a mistake is definitely not the same as total failure.*
Jumping to conclusions	You take one observation and are sure it has only one implication.	*Since I didn't lose weight this week, trying to lose weight is impossible.*	*People don't lose weight every single week, even if their eating has been exactly the same.*
Negative fortune-telling	You make a negative prediction without recognizing it is not the only possible outcome.	*I won't be able to resist the desserts at the party.*	*No one will force me to eat. I need to prepare myself in advance and use the skills I've learned.*
Positive fortune-telling	You are overly optimistic about the most likely outcome.	*I will be able to eat just one cookie, be satisfied, and stop.*	*History shows me that I almost always want more.*
Discounting the positive	You unreasonably discount your positive actions or qualities.	*It doesn't matter if I've lost a few pounds. I deserve credit only after I've lost all of the weight I need to lose.*	*I deserve credit for every positive action I take.*
Emotional reasoning	You think your thoughts must be true because they *feel* true, even if there is evidence to the contrary.	*Since I feel so hopeless about losing weight, it really must be hopeless.*	*Everyone gets discouraged from time to time. It's normal. I'll only stop losing weight if I decide to stop following the program.*

Thinking Mistakes Chart *(continued)*

Thinking Mistakes	Description	Example	Helpful Response
Labeling	You label yourself (or someone else) in a globally negative way without really considering the whole person.	*I'm bad for overeating today.*	*Of course I'm not bad. I just engaged in some unhelpful eating behaviors.*
Mind reading	You are sure you know what others are thinking, even in the absence of compelling data.	*Everyone will think negatively of me if I eat differently.*	*It's likely that some people will be pleased that I'm losing weight and others won't notice or won't care what I'm eating.*
Self-deluding thinking	You tell yourself things that you really do not believe at other times.	*If I eat standing up, it doesn't count.*	*A calorie is a calorie, no matter how I consume it.*
Dysfunctional (unhelpful) rules	You mandate what you or others must or must not do, without taking circumstances into consideration.	*I can't waste food.*	*It's better to waste food in the trash than in my body.*
Irrelevance	You link two unrelated concepts.	*It's okay to eat because I'm so stressed out.*	*Emotional eating is not okay. I need to tolerate my distress or solve a problem.*
Exaggeration	You make a sweeping statement on the basis of a small set of data.	*I'm totally out of control (of my eating).*	*I ate some food I hadn't planned to. But I can start following my plan again right this moment.*

today's to-do list

Each night, remember to check off each task you've completed. Circle any you didn't do, so you can be aware that you didn't follow the program completely.

☐ I weighed myself.

☐ I read my list of reasons to lose weight (and other Response Cards as needed).

☐ I scheduled exercise and dieting activities on My Daily Schedule.

☐ I measured all of my food.

☐ I ate everything slowly and mindfully while sitting down.

☐ I refrained from overeating.

☐ I filled in my food plan *immediately* after eating.

☐ I said NO CHOICE to food that I wasn't supposed to eat.

☐ I stayed within my allotted units (calories, carbs, assigned points).

☐ I exercised (for at least 5 to 30 minutes).

☐ I used distraction techniques when I was hungry or having a craving.

☐ I contacted my diet coach if I needed help.

☐ I was alert for "fooling myself" thoughts.

☐ I used the *Oh, well* technique to deal with disappointment (if needed).

☐ I filled in My Daily Food Plan Chart (page 151) for tomorrow's meals.

☐ I gave myself credit for these things and for: _____

_____

_____

_____

_____

_____.

journal:

What did I do today to avoid unplanned eating? _____

_____

_____

_____

If I deviated, what happened? _____

_____

_____

_____

What sabotaging thoughts did I have? _____

_____

_____

_____

What thinking mistakes did I make? _____

_____

_____

_____

What can I learn from this for next time? _____

_____

_____

_____

Reflections: _____

_____

_____

_____

_____

My Daily Schedule

Use this chart to plan your diet and exercise activities for today.

Time	Activity
6:00 a.m.	
6:30	
7:00	
7:30	
8:00	
8:30	
9:00	
9:30	
10:00	
10:30	
11:00	
11:30	
Noon	
12:30 p.m.	
1:00	
1:30	
2:00	
2:30	
3:00	
3:30	
4:00	
4:30	
5:00	
5:30	
6:00	
6:30	
7:00	
7:30	
8:00	
8:30	
9:00	
9:30	
10:00	
10:30	
11:00	

My Daily Food Plan Chart

units allowed: _____ calories/carbs/assigned points

	Planned Eating Fill In Day Before and Check Off Immediately After Eating				Unplanned Eating Add Immediately After Eating		
	List Food	Amount	Units (calories, carbs, assigned points)	☑	List Food	Amount	Units (calories, carbs, assigned points)
breakfast							
snack							
lunch							
snack							
dinner							
snack							

units consumed: _____ calories/carbs/assigned points

day 27

Respond to Sabotaging Thoughts

You can answer back your sabotaging thoughts by asking yourself certain questions. A dieter I counseled needed to ask herself these questions when she stepped on the scale one day and saw that she had gained a pound. She immediately thought, *This is terrible! I'm failing! I'll never be able to lose weight.* Fortunately, she was able to turn around her thinking by answering these seven questions:

1. What kind of error in thinking could I be making? *Negative fortune-telling*

2. What evidence do I have that the thought is true or untrue? *There have been weeks in the past when I gained a little weight, but I always started losing again.*

3. Is there another way to view this situation? What is it? *It's possible I didn't lose weight this week due to hormonal changes or natural fluctuations.*

4. What is the most realistic outcome of this situation? *If I keep doing what I'm doing, my weight loss will resume.*

5. What is the effect of my believing this thought and what could be the effect of changing my thinking? *If I keep thinking I can't lose weight, I'm likely to become discouraged and abandon my diet. If I change my thinking, I'll keep going.*

6. What advice would I give a friend or family member in the same situation? *I would tell my sister that of course she can lose weight. She just has to have faith and stay on track.*

7. What should I do now? *Read my Response Cards, get reinvigorated, and continue on my diet. Call my diet coach if I need motivation.*

Prepare for sabotaging thoughts that aren't already addressed on one of your Response Cards by doing the following:

☐ Copy the seven questions onto cardstock paper. Carry the list wherever you go so you can respond effectively to your unhelpful thinking.

the seven question technique

1. What kind of thinking error could I be making? (Review the chart on pages 146–147 to help you figure out the answer to this question.)

2. What evidence is there that this thought is true or untrue?

3. Is there another way to view this situation? What is it?

4. What is the most realistic outcome of this situation?

5. What is the effect of my believing this thought and what could be the effect of changing my thinking?

6. What would I tell [a close friend or family member] if he/she were in this situation and had this thought?

7. What should I do now?

what are you thinking?

Sabotaging Thought: I'm not sure I can learn to change my sabotaging thinking. It's so convincing at the moment.

Helpful Response: This is like any other skill. I just have to practice and practice ahead of time so that I'll be able to use this skill when I need it.

today's to-do list

Each night, remember to check off each task you've completed. Circle any you didn't do, so you can be aware that you didn't follow the program completely.

☐ I weighed myself.

☐ I read my list of reasons to lose weight (and other Response Cards as needed).

☐ I scheduled exercise and dieting activities on My Daily Schedule.

☐ I measured all of my food.

☐ I ate everything slowly and mindfully while sitting down.

☐ I refrained from overeating.

☐ I filled in my food plan *immediately* after eating.

☐ I said NO CHOICE to food that I wasn't supposed to eat.

☐ I stayed within my allotted units (calories, carbs, assigned points).

☐ I exercised (for at least 5 to 30 minutes).

☐ I used distraction techniques when I was hungry or having a craving.

☐ I contacted my diet coach if I needed help.

☐ I was alert for "fooling myself" thoughts.

☐ I used the *Oh, well* technique to deal with disappointment (if needed).

☐ I filled in My Daily Food Plan Chart (page 157) for tomorrow's meals.

☐ I gave myself credit for these things and for: _____

_____

_____

_____

_____

_____ .

journal:

What did I do today to avoid unplanned eating? _____

_____

_____

_____

If I deviated, what happened? _____

_____

_____

_____

What sabotaging thoughts did I have? _____

_____

_____

_____

How did I answer back to them? _____

_____

_____

_____

What can I learn from this for next time? _____

_____

_____

_____

Reflections: _____

_____

_____

_____

_____

My Daily Schedule

Use this chart to plan your diet and exercise activities for today.

Time	Activity
6:00 a.m.	
6:30	
7:00	
7:30	
8:00	
8:30	
9:00	
9:30	
10:00	
10:30	
11:00	
11:30	
Noon	
12:30 p.m.	
1:00	
1:30	
2:00	
2:30	
3:00	
3:30	
4:00	
4:30	
5:00	
5:30	
6:00	
6:30	
7:00	
7:30	
8:00	
8:30	
9:00	
9:30	
10:00	
10:30	
11:00	

My Daily Food Plan Chart

units allowed: _____ calories/carbs/assigned points

	Planned Eating Fill In Day Before and Check Off Immediately After Eating				**Unplanned Eating** Add Immediately After Eating		
	List Food	**Amount**	**Units** (calories, carbs, assigned points)	☑	**List Food**	**Amount**	**Units** (calories, carbs, assigned points)
breakfast							
snack							
lunch							
snack							
dinner							
snack							

units consumed: _____ calories/carbs/assigned points

day 28

Prepare for Another Weigh-In

Okay, you've made it through another week of dieting on the Beck Diet Solution program! Tomorrow, you're going to mark the change in your weight on My Weight-Loss Graph on page 127. Get yourself ready by doing the following:

☐ Don't even *think* about skimping on your diet today so that the number on the scale looks better tomorrow. If you do, you'll be giving yourself unhelpful messages: that it's okay to be loose during the week because you'll make up for it all on one day or that starving yourself is acceptable. The goal of the Beck Diet Solution is to help normalize eating patterns every single day—for the rest of your life—which means never overeating or undereating. If your weight goes up this week because you've made mistakes in your eating, face your problems squarely and then solve them.

☐ Make sure your expectations are reasonable. Read Response Card #19 ("Celebrate!"). Remember that most people lose between ½ pound and 2 pounds per week during most weeks. *You will likely lose less weight this week than last* because part of last week's loss was from water. So get yourself mentally prepared to have a smaller weight loss tomorrow. It's perfectly normal.

You also need to know that your weight could go up on any given day or week, *even if you've been following your diet and exercise plans precisely,* due to hormonal or other biological factors. So if you've been doing everything right, don't think it's a catastrophe if the number on the scale doesn't go down this week. Read Response Card #22 ("Be Realistic"). You'll probably lose more next week. If you don't, you can consider cutting your calories or adding in more exercise at that time.

what are you thinking?

Sabotaging Thought: I've worked really hard. If I don't lose a lot of weight, I'll be too discouraged to continue dieting.

Helpful Response: It's highly unlikely that I'll lose a lot of weight in one week. I need to adjust my expectations. If I wanted to become a body builder and put in a lot of hard work for the first two weeks, I wouldn't expect to see huge muscles developing right away. Dieting is hard work, but it will get much easier soon. And if I want all the benefits of losing weight, I have to accept a slow rate of weight loss.

today's to-do list

Each night, remember to check off each task you've completed. Circle any you didn't do, so you can be aware that you didn't follow the program completely.

☐ I weighed myself.

☐ I read my list of reasons to lose weight (and other Response Cards as needed).

☐ I scheduled exercise and dieting activities on My Daily Schedule.

☐ I measured all of my food.

☐ I ate everything slowly and mindfully while sitting down.

☐ I refrained from overeating.

☐ I filled in my food plan *immediately* after eating.

☐ I said NO CHOICE to food that I wasn't supposed to eat.

☐ I stayed within my allotted units (calories, carbs, assigned points).

☐ I exercised (for at least 5 to 30 minutes).

☐ I used distraction techniques when I was hungry or having a craving.

☐ I contacted my diet coach if I needed help.

☐ I was alert for "fooling myself" thoughts.

☐ I used the *Oh, well* technique to deal with disappointment (if needed).

☐ I mentally prepared for weighing in tomorrow.

☐ I filled in My Daily Food Plan Chart (page 163) for tomorrow's meals.

☐ I gave myself credit for these things and for: _____

_____

_____

_____

_____

_____ .

journal:

What did I do today to avoid unplanned eating? _____

_____

_____

_____

If I deviated, what happened? _____

_____

_____

_____

What sabotaging thoughts did I have? _____

_____

_____

_____

How did I answer back to them? _____

_____

_____

_____

What can I learn from this for next time? _____

_____

_____

_____

Reflections: _____

_____

_____

_____

_____

_____

My Daily Schedule

Use this chart to plan your diet and exercise activities for today.

Time	Activity
6:00 a.m.	
6:30	
7:00	
7:30	
8:00	
8:30	
9:00	
9:30	
10:00	
10:30	
11:00	
11:30	
Noon	
12:30 p.m.	
1:00	
1:30	
2:00	
2:30	
3:00	
3:30	
4:00	
4:30	
5:00	
5:30	
6:00	
6:30	
7:00	
7:30	
8:00	
8:30	
9:00	
9:30	
10:00	
10:30	
11:00	

My Daily Food Plan Chart

units allowed: _____ calories/carbs/assigned points

	Planned Eating — Fill In Day Before and Check Off Immediately After Eating				Unplanned Eating — Add Immediately After Eating		
	List Food	Amount	Units (calories, carbs, assigned points)	☑	List Food	Amount	Units (calories, carbs, assigned points)
breakfast							
snack							
lunch							
snack							
dinner							
snack							

units consumed: _____ calories/carbs/assigned points

chapter 9

Week 5

Solve Real-life Problems

Has dieting been relatively easy up till now? This week, I want you to continue getting ready to face potential difficulties. Most of the problems we have dealt with up until this point have been *internal,* concerned mostly with your thoughts and reactions. But you don't diet in a vacuum. You interact with friends, coworkers, and family members—who may react to your dieting efforts in different ways.

In addition, you have places to go and things to do—many of which involve exposure to food and drink that's not on your plan. So this week we focus primarily on *external* challenges and real-life situations in which you have to solve problems related to food and other people, events, and circumstances beyond your control. This week, you will learn how to live your life on a diet.

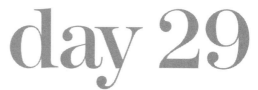

day 29

Say No to Food Pushers

When you weigh yourself this morning, record your change in weight on My Weight-Loss Graph on page 127. If you've lost more than 5 pounds, congratulations! You'll need to start using the graph on page 246. Don't forget to call your diet coach to report your change in weight.

Today, we need to talk about food pushers: people who urge you to eat something that's not on your diet. They fall into three categories:

1. People who are just trying to be nice but don't care whether or not you eat what they offer

2. People who genuinely want you to eat something and are offended if you turn them down

3. People who are deliberately trying to get you to eat something they know isn't on your diet

When people offer you food that you haven't planned to eat, do the following:

☐ Thank them nicely: "Oh, thanks very much, but no thanks."

☐ If appropriate, if the food won't be too tempting, *and if you want to,* you can ask if you can take it with you: "That looks good. Would you mind if I took it home and had it later?" Then add it to your food plan for tomorrow or for some other day.

☐ If they insist, you can give a simple explanation if you want: "Thanks, but I have to watch what I'm eating these days." Or you can just say more firmly, but still politely, "No, thanks. I'm going to pass."

Don't let their reaction impact your decision. Read Response Card #4 ("It's Okay to Disappoint People"). Develop the attitude that *you are completely entitled* to make good food decisions for yourself. Here's what I'd like you to do right now:

☐ Read Response Cards #5 ("Say No to Extra Food") and #14 ("It's Not Okay").

☐ Think about the next couple of people who might try to push food on you. Then ask yourself these questions:

  • Is it reasonable for them to have a strong negative reaction?

  • How long will they be upset? How soon will they actually be thinking about something else?

- What's the worst that will happen if I turn them down? If that happened, what could I say to them?

- If I had to be on a diet because I had a heart condition, wouldn't I refuse what they were offering? Why isn't my goal of losing weight also legitimate?

Now, think about the costs you will incur if you say yes to these food pushers. Check off all the statements below that apply to you:

☐ I'll have to deviate from my plan.

☐ Eating this might set off cravings.

☐ I'll feel like I'm being controlled.

☐ I'll feel weak.

☐ I'll be giving the message that it's okay to push food on me.

☐ I'll feel bad after I eat it.

If you still feel uneasy about turning down a food pusher or you don't feel entitled to say anything, discuss this problem with your diet coach. I'm sure your coach will give you guidance and permission to do what's right for you.

what are you thinking?

Sabotaging Thought: If I don't eat, [this food pusher] will be upset.

Helpful Response: She may not be as upset as I fear, but even if she is, so what? I should turn down any food I hadn't planned to eat. I'm entitled to do this as long as I'm politely assertive. I shouldn't let her push me around.

today's to-do list

Each night, remember to check off each task you've completed. Circle any you didn't do, so you can be aware that you didn't follow the program completely.

☐ I weighed myself, recorded it on My Weight-Loss Graph, and reported the change to my diet coach.

☐ I read my list of reasons to lose weight (and other Response Cards as needed).

☐ I scheduled exercise and dieting activities on My Daily Schedule.

☐ I measured all of my food.

☐ I ate everything slowly and mindfully while sitting down.

☐ I refrained from overeating.

☐ I filled in my food plan *immediately* after eating.

☐ I said NO CHOICE to food that I wasn't supposed to eat.

☐ I stayed within my allotted units (calories, carbs, assigned points).

☐ I exercised (for at least 5 to 30 minutes).

☐ I used distraction techniques when I was hungry or having a craving.

☐ I was alert for "fooling myself" thoughts.

☐ I used the *Oh, well* technique to deal with disappointment (if needed).

☐ I prepared myself mentally for dealing with food pushers.

☐ I filled in My Daily Food Plan Chart (page 170) for tomorrow's meals.

☐ I gave myself credit for these things and for: _____

_____

_____

_____

_____

_____ .

journal:

What did I do today to avoid unplanned eating? _____

_____

_____

_____

If I deviated, what happened? _____

_____

_____

_____

What sabotaging thoughts did I have? _____

_____

_____

_____

How did I answer back to them? _____

_____

_____

_____

What can I learn from this for next time? _____

_____

_____

_____

Reflections: _____

_____

_____

_____

_____

My Daily Schedule

Use this chart to plan your diet and exercise activities for today.

Time	Activity
6:00 a.m.	
6:30	
7:00	
7:30	
8:00	
8:30	
9:00	
9:30	
10:00	
10:30	
11:00	
11:30	
Noon	
12:30 p.m.	
1:00	
1:30	
2:00	
2:30	
3:00	
3:30	
4:00	
4:30	
5:00	
5:30	
6:00	
6:30	
7:00	
7:30	
8:00	
8:30	
9:00	
9:30	
10:00	
10:30	
11:00	

My Daily Food Plan Chart

units allowed: _____ calories/carbs/assigned points

	Planned Eating — Fill In Day Before and Check Off Immediately After Eating				Unplanned Eating — Add Immediately After Eating		
	List Food	Amount	Units (calories, carbs, assigned points)	☑	List Food	Amount	Units (calories, carbs, assigned points)
breakfast							
snack							
lunch							
snack							
dinner							
snack							

units consumed: _____ calories/carbs/assigned points

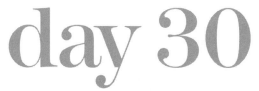

day 30

Eat Out with Ease

It's important for you to fully engage in life and to enjoy going to restaurants, parties, celebrations, special holiday feasts, and other people's houses for meals. You just need to develop helpful attitudes and have a plan of action. The next time one of these situations arises, do the following:

☐ Decide in advance how many calories (or carbs or assigned points) you are going to have when you eat out. It's okay to eat a little less food earlier in the day so you can eat a little bit more at this meal. Or it's fine to decide that you're going to eat 25 to 50 percent more than you usually do at a particular meal. For example, if you usually eat a 600-calorie dinner, plan instead to eat 750 to 900 calories. Many people can do this once a week without having the extra amount show up on the scale—however, some people can't. You'll need to see what works for you.

☐ Before you go out, read your list of reasons to lose weight and review all of your relevant Response Cards.

☐ If you plan to eat at a restaurant, check if they post their menu on their Web site. Decide before you go what—as well as how much—you're going to eat and then calculate the number of calories, carbs, or assigned points your meal will have. Making decisions in advance is much safer than making split-second decisions once you're out and presented with a lot of food choices.

☐ If you can't find out what kinds of foods will be served, survey the offerings when you get to the venue. Decide what—and how much—you can eat while staying within your parameters. You will likely have to skip hors d'oeuvres, bread, and dessert, and eat just part of the main course.

☐ If you're going to a party or dinner in a private home, offer to bring something you *can* eat, such as steamed or raw vegetables, salsa, a low-calorie soup, salad, or fruit.

☐ Don't be reluctant to make special requests at a restaurant or catered affair.

☐ When your food arrives, portion off the amount you planned to have and push the rest of the food to the side of your plate or transfer it to a bread plate.

☐ When you've finished eating, if you're tempted to eat more, excuse yourself, go to the rest-room or step outside, and read your Response Cards again. Or try such techniques as putting your napkin on your plate, asking to have your leftover food wrapped up immediately, or pushing your plate toward the center of the table.

☐ During holidays, you can decide to increase your calories by 100 to 300 calories per day, knowing that you could gain a pound or two. However, don't gain weight because you've just allowed yourself to get looser with your eating. Make sure to plan what you're going to eat in advance and monitor what you eat and drink. As soon as the holidays are over, go back to your usual calorie limit. Keep weighing yourself every day, though, and even if it's in the middle of the holiday season, return to your usual calorie limit if you go up by 3 pounds.

Now, how are you going to get yourself to do these things? You may need an attitude transplant. The attitude you develop toward eating out may very well predict your future success. Here's when I know dieters have really turned the corner and will be able to keep losing weight and keep it off: when they tell me they leave a special event or a restaurant and say to themselves, *I'm so glad I didn't overeat!* Instead of feeling deprived, they feel really good that they stuck to their plan.

what are you thinking?

Sabotaging Thought: I should be able to enjoy myself at special occasions.

Helpful Response: Eating differently doesn't mean I can't enjoy other aspects of this occasion. But I have to face the fact that I may not get as much enjoyment from food as I used to. Since I'll be faced with many special occasions in my lifetime, I have a choice: I can eat whatever I want OR I can be thinner. But I can't have it both ways.

today's to-do list

Each night, remember to check off each task you've completed. Circle any you didn't do, so you can be aware that you didn't follow the program completely.

☐ I weighed myself.

☐ I read my list of reasons to lose weight (and other Response Cards as needed).

☐ I scheduled exercise and dieting activities on My Daily Schedule.

☐ I measured all of my food.

☐ I ate everything slowly and mindfully while sitting down.

☐ I refrained from overeating.

☐ I filled in my food plan *immediately* after eating.

☐ I said NO CHOICE to food that I wasn't supposed to eat.

☐ I stayed within my allotted units (calories, carbs, assigned points).

☐ I exercised (for at least 5 to 30 minutes).

☐ I used distraction techniques when I was hungry or having a craving.

☐ I contacted my diet coach if I needed help.

☐ I was alert for "fooling myself" thoughts.

☐ I used the *Oh, well* technique to deal with disappointment (if needed).

☐ I created a plan for the next time I eat out.

☐ I filled in My Daily Food Plan Chart (page 176) for tomorrow's meals.

☐ I gave myself credit for these things and for: _____

_____

_____

_____

_____ .

journal:

What did I do today to avoid unplanned eating? _____

_____

_____

_____

If I deviated, what happened? _____

_____

_____

_____

What sabotaging thoughts did I have? _____

_____

_____

_____

How did I answer back to them? _____

_____

_____

_____

What can I learn from this for next time? _____

_____

_____

_____

Reflections: _____

_____

_____

_____

_____

My Daily Schedule

Use this chart to plan your diet and exercise activities for today.

Time	Activity
6:00 a.m.	
6:30	
7:00	
7:30	
8:00	
8:30	
9:00	
9:30	
10:00	
10:30	
11:00	
11:30	
Noon	
12:30 p.m.	
1:00	
1:30	
2:00	
2:30	
3:00	
3:30	
4:00	
4:30	
5:00	
5:30	
6:00	
6:30	
7:00	
7:30	
8:00	
8:30	
9:00	
9:30	
10:00	
10:30	
11:00	

My Daily Food Plan Chart

units allowed: _____ calories/carbs/assigned points

	Planned Eating Fill In Day Before and Check Off Immediately After Eating				Unplanned Eating Add Immediately After Eating		
	List Food	**Amount**	**Units** (calories, carbs, assigned points)	☑	**List Food**	**Amount**	**Units** (calories, carbs, assigned points)
breakfast							
snack							
lunch							
snack							
dinner							
snack							

units consumed: _____ calories/carbs/assigned points

date: _____

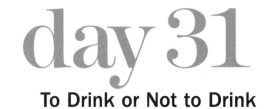

day 31

To Drink or Not to Drink

Drinking alcohol is a personal choice. You may prefer wine, a mixed drink, or a beer to a food-related treat. Or maybe you're more like me: You'd rather spend calories on food than on drinks. What does your diet say about drinking? Are you allowed alcohol? How often? How much?

Alcohol calories add up fast if you aren't careful, especially when you are out at dinner or at a party. You have to learn to plan your alcohol intake before you go, just as you do your food intake. Don't decide on the spur of the moment to have a drink—or an extra drink. Really solidify your ability to make and to follow a plan.

If you plan to have a drink, here's what I want you to do:

☐ Sip slowly and savor every sip.

☐ Be careful! Alcohol loosens inhibitions, and you may give in to temptation, resulting in unplanned eating and/or drinking.

☐ Beware of friends or family members who push you to drink more. Read Response Card #4 ("It's Okay to Disappoint People") and review Day 29 (pages 165–170) before you go because you can deal with "alcohol pushers" in the same way you deal with food pushers.

☐ Make a commitment now to drink moderately so you won't have to cut back too much on eating. Remember, if your diet isn't healthy and balanced, your body will rebel and you'll surely start to gain back weight.

what are you thinking?

Sabotaging Thought: It's sad that I have to forgo a glass of my favorite wine with dinner.

Helpful Response: I don't have to give up wine entirely. I can modify my diet plan as long as I stay within its parameters (calories, carbs, or assigned points). I'll just have to make sure the other calories I eat count so that I get the proper nutrition for the day.

today's to-do list

Each night, remember to check off each task you've completed. Circle any you didn't do, so you can be aware that you didn't follow the program completely.

☐ I weighed myself.

☐ I read my list of reasons to lose weight (and other Response Cards as needed).

☐ I scheduled exercise and dieting activities on My Daily Schedule.

☐ I measured all of my food.

☐ I ate everything slowly and mindfully while sitting down.

☐ I refrained from overeating.

☐ I filled in my food plan *immediately* after eating.

☐ I said NO CHOICE to food that I wasn't supposed to eat.

☐ I stayed within my allotted units (calories, carbs, assigned points).

☐ I exercised (for at least 5 to 30 minutes).

☐ I used distraction techniques when I was hungry or having a craving.

☐ I contacted my diet coach if I needed help.

☐ I was alert for "fooling myself" thoughts.

☐ I used the *Oh, well* technique to deal with disappointment (if needed).

☐ I created a plan for drinking alcohol.

☐ I filled in My Daily Food Plan Chart (page 181) for tomorrow's meals.

☐ I gave myself credit for these things and for: _____

_____

_____

_____

_____

_____ .

journal:

What did I do today to avoid unplanned eating? _____

_____

_____

_____

If I deviated, what happened?_____

_____

_____

_____

What sabotaging thoughts did I have?_____

_____

_____

_____

How did I answer back to them? _____

_____

_____

_____

What can I learn from this for next time? _____

_____

_____

_____

Reflections: _____

_____

_____

_____

_____

My Daily Schedule

Use this chart to plan your diet and exercise activities for today.

Time	Activity
6:00 a.m.	
6:30	
7:00	
7:30	
8:00	
8:30	
9:00	
9:30	
10:00	
10:30	
11:00	
11:30	
Noon	
12:30 p.m.	
1:00	
1:30	
2:00	
2:30	
3:00	
3:30	
4:00	
4:30	
5:00	
5:30	
6:00	
6:30	
7:00	
7:30	
8:00	
8:30	
9:00	
9:30	
10:00	
10:30	
11:00	

My Daily Food Plan Chart

units allowed: _____ calories/carbs/assigned points

	Planned Eating — Fill In Day Before and Check Off Immediately After Eating				**Unplanned Eating** — Add Immediately After Eating		
	List Food	**Amount**	**Units** (calories, carbs, assigned points)	☑	**List Food**	**Amount**	**Units** (calories, carbs, assigned points)
breakfast							
snack							
lunch							
snack							
dinner							
snack							

units consumed: _____ calories/carbs/assigned points

day 32

Take It on the Road

Many dieters are anxious about traveling. They don't know what kinds of foods will be available; whether they'll be able to stick to their diet when they don't have control over the food that's served; and whether they will be able to resist temptations to eat unplanned food.

There are several strategies you can use when traveling to avoid undoing all of the good work you have done so far. First of all, you need to realize that it may be unrealistic—as well as unreasonable—to follow your usual plan to the letter while traveling. This doesn't mean you should abandon your plan altogether, of course. Instead, come up with a time-limited variation of the plan you've been following to implement while traveling.

Decide before you go how many extra calories you're going to allow yourself, either each day or for the entire time you're away. It's perfectly reasonable to say to yourself, *Okay, I'm going away on a trip ... I'm going to want to have a drink every night or to enjoy small portions of the local specialties ... I'm going to have up to an extra 300 calories every day I'm away, which means I may gain a pound or two ... I'll lose it when I return home by getting back to my usual diet and exercise plans.*

To develop a strategy, think about your next trip:

- Where are you going? _____

- How long will you be away? _____

- If you're not careful, how much weight do you think you could gain? _____ pounds

- How much control will you have over available food? _____

- Can you arrange to have access to a refrigerator or microwave? ☐ yes ☐ no

- Can you bring or buy some favorite snack foods? ☐ yes ☐ no

- Who will be with you? _____

- Will they likely support, be neutral, or undermine your efforts? _____

Now, I'd like you to develop a plan for this trip. Check off the most desirable and reasonable option from the choices below:

☐ Continue to eat exactly as you are now.

☐ Continue to eat as you are now but also factor in up to 300 extra calories a day (of food or alcohol). This might be in the form of a piece of bread and butter with dinner, a mixed drink, or a slice of cake, for example.

☐ Continue to eat as you are now but on two or three days also factor in minor splurges of up to 500 extra calories. These extra calories could come from two glasses of wine and an appetizer, sampling small amounts of several different local specialties, or a special dessert.

☐ Continue to eat as you are now but also factor in up to 1,000 extra calories one time only (preferably on your last day, so you have something to look forward to). This might come from a dinner with larger portions and either an alcoholic drink, an appetizer, bread, or a dessert.

Make sure to take this workbook and all your Response Cards with you. You may find you need to read them more often than usual. Reread Days 30 and 31 (pages 171–181) to refresh your strategies for eating out and drinking alcohol. Also, try to incorporate additional exercise while away from home. You can inquire before you go about the availability of a gym, running track, bike rental, swimming pool, or other exercise opportunities. And try walking to places of interest—often the best way to explore a new location is on foot.

On your way home, get re-energized for going back to your usual eating plan. Recognize that if you gained a pound or two, you'll probably lose it within the next two weeks—no long-term harm done. Plan what you're going to eat that day and the next. Think about when you're going to the grocery store and when you're going to prepare your meals. And don't forget to get right back on your exercise program, too.

what are you thinking?

Sabotaging Thought: I know I won't have control over my food. What if everything I'm served is really high in calories?

Helpful Response: I might be able to request food that fits in my plan. If not, I'll just have to eat smaller portions and eat even more slowly and mindfully than usual. The worst that will happen is that I'll be hungry sometimes. But I've already proven to myself that I can tolerate hunger. And I'll be so happy that I limited my eating when I come home and get on the scale.

today's to-do list

Each night, remember to check off each task you've completed. Circle any you didn't do, so you can be aware that you didn't follow the program completely.

☐ I weighed myself.

☐ I read my list of reasons to lose weight (and other Response Cards as needed).

☐ I scheduled exercise and dieting activities on My Daily Schedule.

☐ I measured all of my food.

☐ I ate everything slowly and mindfully while sitting down.

☐ I refrained from overeating.

☐ I filled in my food plan *immediately* after eating.

☐ I said NO CHOICE to food that I wasn't supposed to eat.

☐ I stayed within my allotted units (calories, carbs, assigned points).

☐ I exercised (for at least 5 to 30 minutes).

☐ I used distraction techniques when I was hungry or having a craving.

☐ I contacted my diet coach if I needed help.

☐ I was alert for "fooling myself" thoughts.

☐ I used the *Oh, well* technique to deal with disappointment (if needed).

☐ I created a plan for the next time I travel.

☐ I filled in My Daily Food Plan Chart (page 187) for tomorrow's meals.

☐ I gave myself credit for these things and for: _____

_____

_____

_____

_____

_____.

journal:

What did I do today to avoid unplanned eating? _____

_____

_____

_____

If I deviated, what happened? _____

_____

_____

_____

What sabotaging thoughts did I have? _____

_____

_____

_____

How did I answer back to them? _____

_____

_____

_____

What can I learn from this for next time? _____

_____

_____

_____

Reflections: _____

_____

_____

_____

_____

My Daily Schedule

Use this chart to plan your diet and exercise activities for today.

Time	Activity
6:00 a.m.	
6:30	
7:00	
7:30	
8:00	
8:30	
9:00	
9:30	
10:00	
10:30	
11:00	
11:30	
Noon	
12:30 p.m.	
1:00	
1:30	
2:00	
2:30	
3:00	
3:30	
4:00	
4:30	
5:00	
5:30	
6:00	
6:30	
7:00	
7:30	
8:00	
8:30	
9:00	
9:30	
10:00	
10:30	
11:00	

My Daily Food Plan Chart

units allowed: _____ calories/carbs/assigned points

	Planned Eating Fill In Day Before and Check Off Immediately After Eating				Unplanned Eating Add Immediately After Eating		
	List Food	Amount	Units (calories, carbs, assigned points)	☑	List Food	Amount	Units (calories, carbs, assigned points)
breakfast							
snack							
lunch							
snack							
dinner							
snack							

units consumed: _____ calories/carbs/assigned points

day 33

Soothe Your Emotions Without Food

At one time or another, most dieters eat for emotional reasons. They think, *Because I'm upset, I have to eat.* But people who don't struggle with dieting don't generally eat in response to feeling distressed.

Here's what to do when you're tempted to soothe yourself with food and can't directly solve your problem or respond to the thoughts that are causing the distress. Read this list now, return to it whenever you need it, and check off each item as you complete it:

☐ Identify your negative emotions and distinguish them from the feeling of hunger. For example, recognize that you're upset because your mother criticized you, you're anxious because there's a problem with your child, or you're just bored or at loose ends.

☐ Say NO CHOICE. Tell yourself that you need to learn the habit of refraining from eating in response to negative emotions or you will be at risk for regaining any weight you've lost.

☐ Recognize that food may comfort you, but THE EFFECT IS ONLY TEMPORARY. Afterwards, you'll feel worse. If you don't give in, you'll feel better and more in control.

☐ Change your focus. Try at least five things on My Distraction Techniques Chart (pages 76–77).

☐ Have a cup of tea.

☐ Practice relaxation techniques: deep breathing, stretching, and counting slowly to 10. You can do these almost anywhere, even in a restroom if need be.

☐ Tolerate your distress. Prove to yourself that the experience of negative emotions is uncomfortable, but nothing "bad" will happen if you just let yourself feel the feelings. In fact, you'll learn something important: You never need to eat just because you're feeling upset.

☐ Read Response Card #23 ("Don't Comfort Myself with Food") as often as needed.

what are you thinking?

Sabotaging Thought: Eating is my only comfort.

Helpful Response: I certainly could comfort myself in other ways. Now, I have to decide: I can eat when I'm upset and gain weight OR I can learn to tolerate negative emotions (or soothe myself by doing something else) and get—and stay—thinner.

today's to-do list

Each night, remember to check off each task you've completed. Circle any you didn't do, so you can be aware that you didn't follow the program completely.

☐ I weighed myself.

☐ I read my list of reasons to lose weight (and other Response Cards as needed).

☐ I scheduled exercise and dieting activities on My Daily Schedule.

☐ I measured all of my food.

☐ I ate everything slowly and mindfully while sitting down.

☐ I refrained from overeating.

☐ I filled in my food plan *immediately* after eating.

☐ I said NO CHOICE to food that I wasn't supposed to eat.

☐ I stayed within my allotted units (calories, carbs, assigned points).

☐ I exercised (for at least 5 to 30 minutes).

☐ I used distraction techniques when I was hungry or having a craving.

☐ I contacted my diet coach if I needed help.

☐ I was alert for "fooling myself" thoughts.

☐ I used the *Oh, well* technique to deal with disappointment (if needed).

☐ I created a plan for the next time I'm upset.

☐ I filled in My Daily Food Plan Chart (page 193) for tomorrow's meals.

☐ I gave myself credit for these things and for: _____

_____

_____

_____

_____

_____ .

journal:

What did I do today to avoid unplanned eating? _____

_____

_____

_____

If I deviated, what happened? _____

_____

_____

_____

What sabotaging thoughts did I have? _____

_____

_____

_____

How did I answer back to them? _____

_____

_____

_____

What can I learn from this for next time? _____

_____

_____

_____

Reflections: _____

_____

_____

_____

_____

My Daily Schedule

Use this chart to plan your diet and exercise activities for today.

Time	Activity
6:00 a.m.	
6:30	
7:00	
7:30	
8:00	
8:30	
9:00	
9:30	
10:00	
10:30	
11:00	
11:30	
Noon	
12:30 p.m.	
1:00	
1:30	
2:00	
2:30	
3:00	
3:30	
4:00	
4:30	
5:00	
5:30	
6:00	
6:30	
7:00	
7:30	
8:00	
8:30	
9:00	
9:30	
10:00	
10:30	
11:00	

My Daily Food Plan Chart

units allowed: _____ calories/carbs/assigned points

	Planned Eating Fill In Day Before and Check Off Immediately After Eating				**Unplanned Eating** Add Immediately After Eating		
	List Food	Amount	Units (calories, carbs, assigned points)	☑	List Food	Amount	Units (calories, carbs, assigned points)
breakfast							
snack							
lunch							
snack							
dinner							
snack							

units consumed: _____ calories/carbs/assigned points

day 34

Do Problem Solving

It's beyond the scope of this workbook to solve the many and varied problems that life invariably brings. But you *can* use problem-solving strategies when circumstances are in your control and coping strategies when they're not to minimize the chances of eating in response to these difficulties.

Many dieters I've worked with have experienced a number of significant life problems: They have separated from spouses or partners. They have encountered relationship difficulties with children, parents, extended family members, and friends. They have had serious medical issues. Some have had family members who became ill and died. They have lost jobs. They have had financial reverses. *And they have learned to cope with all of these events without turning to food for comfort.*

It was obviously inappropriate to try to "solve" some problems, such as the profound loss some experienced when a family member died. I could—and did—offer a sympathetic ear and a shoulder to cry on. I also encouraged them to lean on others at such times and to ask for support. But many dieters had problems that *could* be solved or at least partially solved.

If the difficulty you're experiencing is under your control, follow the sequence I used with a woman I counseled when she was frustrated with her school-aged children.

☐ **Define the problem specifically.** It was hard for us to solve the global problem: "My kids are out of control." It was easier for us to solve the problem once we broke it down: "I can't get the kids to clean their rooms, do their homework, help with the dishes, and stop fighting with each other."

☐ **See what goes through your mind when you think about the problem. Are you having thoughts that could get in the way of problem solving?** My patient thought, "My kids are bad; they shouldn't act that way." Her thinking undermined her creativity and motivation to solve the problem.

☐ **Respond to unhelpful thinking with the seven question technique from page 153.** When my patient asked herself these questions, she concluded: "Even though my kids are doing these things, I guess they're not 'bad.' They do *some* of the things I ask. They're undisciplined because I haven't known which strategies to use with them. If I learn what to do, they'll probably respond. If I view them as bad, I'll be angry and upset and won't be very effective. If I realize that I can change what *I* do, I'll feel more in control and probably be more effective. If my friend Sally were in this situation, I'd encourage her to get some help. I guess I should get someone to teach me the skills I need."

☐ **Once you've responded to your interfering thoughts, use the last question—What should I do?—as a spur to brainstorm lots of solutions.** Don't try to go it alone; ask for support. Friends and family members can frequently think of solutions that haven't occurred to you.

☐ **Look at each potential solution, decide which one is best to try first, and then implement it.** Repeat this process with other possible solutions as often as necessary.

what are you thinking?

Sabotaging Thought: I just don't know what to do. I really feel like eating.

Helpful Response: Reach out for help! Eating will distract you only temporarily. You'll have to face the problem sooner or later. Might as well try to solve it now.

today's to-do list

Each night, remember to check off each task you've completed. Circle any you didn't do, so you can be aware that you didn't follow the program completely.

☐ I weighed myself.

☐ I read my list of reasons to lose weight (and other Response Cards as needed).

☐ I scheduled exercise and dieting activities on My Daily Schedule.

☐ I measured all of my food.

☐ I ate everything slowly and mindfully while sitting down.

☐ I refrained from overeating.

☐ I filled in my food plan *immediately* after eating.

☐ I said NO CHOICE to food that I wasn't supposed to eat.

☐ I stayed within my allotted units (calories, carbs, assigned points).

☐ I exercised (for at least 5 to 30 minutes).

☐ I used distraction techniques when I was hungry or having a craving.

☐ I contacted my diet coach if I needed help.

☐ I was alert for "fooling myself" thoughts.

☐ I used the *Oh, well* technique to deal with disappointment (if needed).

☐ I created a plan for the next time I have a problem.

☐ I filled in My Daily Food Plan Chart (page 199) for tomorrow's meals.

☐ I gave myself credit for these things and for: _____

_____

_____

_____

_____

_____.

journal:

What did I do today to avoid unplanned eating? _____

_____

_____

_____

If I deviated, what happened? _____

_____

_____

_____

What sabotaging thoughts did I have? _____

_____

_____

_____

How did I answer back to them? _____

_____

_____

_____

What can I learn from this for next time? _____

_____

_____

_____

Reflections: _____

_____

_____

_____

_____

_____

My Daily Schedule

Use this chart to plan your diet and exercise activities for today.

Time	Activity
6:00 a.m.	
6:30	
7:00	
7:30	
8:00	
8:30	
9:00	
9:30	
10:00	
10:30	
11:00	
11:30	
Noon	
12:30 p.m.	
1:00	
1:30	
2:00	
2:30	
3:00	
3:30	
4:00	
4:30	
5:00	
5:30	
6:00	
6:30	
7:00	
7:30	
8:00	
8:30	
9:00	
9:30	
10:00	
10:30	
11:00	

My Daily Food Plan Chart

units allowed: _____ calories/carbs/assigned points

	Planned Eating Fill In Day Before and Check Off Immediately After Eating				Unplanned Eating Add Immediately After Eating		
	List Food	**Amount**	**Units** (calories, carbs, assigned points)	☑	**List Food**	**Amount**	**Units** (calories, carbs, assigned points)
breakfast							
snack							
lunch							
snack							
dinner							
snack							

units consumed: _____ calories/carbs/assigned points

day 35

Prepare for the Scale

Tomorrow marks the beginning of your sixth week using the Beck Diet Solution program. If you have worked through all of the steps in this workbook so far, chances are you have continued to lose excess weight. Before you step on the scale tomorrow morning, remember that the number you see has no moral value. You're not "bad" if the number has gone up.

If you've lost weight this week, great! If not, remember that weight is supposed to fluctuate slightly day to day, just as your blood pressure and temperature do. If you lost weight last week and have kept your food intake and exercise constant, you'll most likely start losing again next week. If you haven't lost weight for two weeks, measure your food more carefully, look for "hidden calories" (especially if you eat out), and cut your calories a little or increase your exercise.

Tomorrow, you will do the following:

☐ Record your change in weight on My Weight-Loss Graph (page 127 or 246).

☐ Consider making a copy of the graph and carrying it with you. This visual reminder of your progress can be quite motivating.

what are you thinking?

Sabotaging Thought: It's hard not to be disappointed by a small loss. I wish I didn't have to diet anymore.

Helpful Response: If I want to keep my weight down forever, I have to accept the fact that I'll always be dieting to some degree. It doesn't matter if I lose slowly because I'm basically going to be eating the same way from now on.

today's to-do list

Each night, remember to check off each task you've completed. Circle any you didn't do, so you can be aware that you didn't follow the program completely.

☐ I weighed myself.

☐ I read my list of reasons to lose weight (and other Response Cards as needed).

☐ I scheduled exercise and dieting activities on My Daily Schedule.

☐ I measured all of my food.

☐ I ate everything slowly and mindfully while sitting down.

☐ I refrained from overeating.

☐ I filled in my food plan *immediately* after eating.

☐ I said NO CHOICE to food that I wasn't supposed to eat.

☐ I stayed within my allotted units (calories, carbs, assigned points).

☐ I exercised (for at least 5 to 30 minutes).

☐ I used distraction techniques when I was hungry or having a craving.

☐ I contacted my diet coach if I needed help.

☐ I was alert for "fooling myself" thoughts.

☐ I used the *Oh, well* technique to deal with disappointment (if needed).

☐ I prepared myself mentally to weigh in tomorrow.

☐ I filled in My Daily Food Plan Chart (page 204) for tomorrow's meals.

☐ I gave myself credit for these things and for: _____

_____

_____

_____

_____

_____.

journal:

What did I do today to avoid unplanned eating? _____

_____

_____

_____

If I deviated, what happened? _____

_____

_____

_____

What sabotaging thoughts did I have? _____

_____

_____

_____

How did I answer back to them? _____

_____

_____

_____

What can I learn from this for next time? _____

_____

_____

_____

Reflections: _____

_____

_____

_____

_____

My Daily Schedule

Use this chart to plan your diet and exercise activities for today.

Time	Activity
6:00 a.m.	
6:30	
7:00	
7:30	
8:00	
8:30	
9:00	
9:30	
10:00	
10:30	
11:00	
11:30	
Noon	
12:30 p.m.	
1:00	
1:30	
2:00	
2:30	
3:00	
3:30	
4:00	
4:30	
5:00	
5:30	
6:00	
6:30	
7:00	
7:30	
8:00	
8:30	
9:00	
9:30	
10:00	
10:30	
11:00	

My Daily Food Plan Chart

units allowed: _____ calories/carbs/assigned points

	Planned Eating Fill In Day Before and Check Off Immediately After Eating				Unplanned Eating Add Immediately After Eating		
	List Food	Amount	Units (calories, carbs, assigned points)	☑	List Food	Amount	Units (calories, carbs, assigned points)
breakfast							
snack							
lunch							
snack							
dinner							
snack							

units consumed: _____ calories/carbs/assigned points

chapter 10

Week 6

Hone Your New Skills

Five weeks have gone by since you first started the Beck Diet Solution program. You have learned many useful tools, such as what to do when you want to eat but know you shouldn't and how to resist food temptations that bombard you every day, at home, on TV, at work—even walking down the street! Doesn't it feel great to know that you can be in control of what you eat, how much you eat, and when you eat? Isn't it a relief not to be at the mercy of internal and external triggers? To know that just because you're hungry, having cravings, or are upset, it doesn't mean you have to eat? Best of all, because you will continue to practice, you're going to have these skills forever.

Last week, we applied the program's skills to real-life situations. This week, you'll learn tools to build your confidence, reduce your overall stress, keep up with exercise, handle weight plateaus, and enrich your life.

day 36

Believe in Yourself

First thing this morning, record your change in weight on My Weight-Loss Graph (page 127 or 246). Call your diet coach and report your progress. Be sure to read Response Card #19 ("Celebrate!") if you've lost weight, Response Card #22 ("Be Realistic") if you haven't but have been faithful to your diet and exercise programs, or Response Card #13 ("Can't Have It Both Ways") if you haven't been sticking to your plans.

At some point, many dieters start to question whether they've really actually changed their relationship with food and whether they'll be able to keep losing weight. I want you to recognize—right now—that the reason you've been successful and will continue to be successful is that you have learned a particular skill set on the Beck Diet Solution program. Do the following:

☐ Build your confidence by checking off the progress you've made on the Believe It Chart on the facing page.

☐ Read this list every morning for as long as it takes for you to believe in yourself and the skills you have learned.

Believe It Chart

I have lost weight (and will be able to keep off excess weight) because I now know how to do these things:

- ☐ Choose a nutritious diet plan.
- ☐ Modify a diet plan (in advance) to suit me and my circumstances.
- ☐ Consistently make time for exercise and all my dieting activities.
- ☐ Arrange my environment for dieting success.
- ☐ Throw away leftover or tempting food.
- ☐ Plan my eating in writing.
- ☐ Eat slowly and mindfully while sitting down.
- ☐ Monitor everything I eat in writing.
- ☐ Tolerate hunger.
- ☐ Avoid or deal effectively with triggers.
- ☐ Resist cravings.
- ☐ Recognize normal fullness.
- ☐ Avoid unplanned eating and overeating.
- ☐ Make myself get on the scale daily.
- ☐ Prepare myself for what the scale will say.
- ☐ Identify and counteract my sabotaging thoughts.
- ☐ Respond to a sense of unfairness.
- ☐ Give myself credit.
- ☐ Squarely face my diet mistakes.
- ☐ Plan how to avoid these mistakes in the future.
- ☐ Get back on track immediately after I stray.
- ☐ Assertively say no to food pushers.
- ☐ Stick to the plan I made for drinking alcohol.
- ☐ Seek out support and ask for help when I need it.
- ☐ Plan for special events and traveling.
- ☐ Cope with negative (and positive) emotions without turning to food.
- ☐ Handle disappointment.
- ☐ Cope with discouragement.
- ☐ Continuously motivate myself to do all of these things.
- ☐ _____
- ☐ _____
- ☐ _____

what are you thinking?

Sabotaging Thought: I'm superstitious: If I start to think this is really working, I might jinx myself.

Helpful Response: Believing in myself can't lead to back luck. In fact, reminding myself of all of the skills I've developed will help me get through the harder times.

today's to-do list

Each night, remember to check off each task you've completed. Circle any you didn't do, so you can be aware that you didn't follow the program completely.

☐ I weighed myself, recorded it on My Weight-Loss Graph, and reported the change to my diet coach.

☐ I read my list of reasons to lose weight (and other Response Cards as needed).

☐ I scheduled exercise and dieting activities on My Daily Schedule.

☐ I measured all of my food.

☐ I ate everything slowly and mindfully while sitting down.

☐ I refrained from overeating.

☐ I filled in my food plan *immediately* after eating.

☐ I said NO CHOICE to food that I wasn't supposed to eat.

☐ I stayed within my allotted units (calories, carbs, assigned points).

☐ I exercised (for at least 5 to 30 minutes).

☐ I used distraction techniques when I was hungry or having a craving.

☐ I was alert for "fooling myself" thoughts.

☐ I used the *Oh, well* technique to deal with disappointment (if needed).

☐ I filled in My Daily Food Plan Chart (page 211) for tomorrow's meals.

☐ I gave myself credit for these things and for: _____

_____

_____

_____

_____

_____ .

journal:

What did I do today to avoid unplanned eating? _____

_____

_____

_____

If I deviated, what happened? _____

_____

_____

_____

What sabotaging thoughts did I have? _____

_____

_____

_____

How did I answer back to them? _____

_____

_____

_____

What can I learn from this for next time? _____

_____

_____

_____

Reflections: _____

_____

_____

_____

_____

My Daily Schedule

Use this chart to plan your diet and exercise activities for today.

Time	Activity
6:00 a.m.	
6:30	
7:00	
7:30	
8:00	
8:30	
9:00	
9:30	
10:00	
10:30	
11:00	
11:30	
Noon	
12:30 p.m.	
1:00	
1:30	
2:00	
2:30	
3:00	
3:30	
4:00	
4:30	
5:00	
5:30	
6:00	
6:30	
7:00	
7:30	
8:00	
8:30	
9:00	
9:30	
10:00	
10:30	
11:00	

My Daily Food Plan Chart

units allowed: _____ calories/carbs/assigned points

	Planned Eating Fill In Day Before and Check Off Immediately After Eating				Unplanned Eating Add Immediately After Eating		
	List Food	Amount	Units (calories, carbs, assigned points)	☑	List Food	Amount	Units (calories, carbs, assigned points)
breakfast							
snack							
lunch							
snack							
dinner							
snack							

units consumed: _____ calories/carbs/assigned points

day 37

De-stress Yourself

Stress is not necessarily bad. Mild stress can motivate us to work harder, to meet a deadline, and to accomplish our goals. However, too much stress—or stress that lasts for long periods—can contribute to overeating. Even if you're feeling pretty good right now, today I want you to learn how to handle stress better. Once you reduce the general stress in your life, maintaining your diet becomes easier.

Practice the following:

☐ **Solve problems.** On Day 34 (pages 194–199), you learned a system for responding to negative thinking in order to solve problems. Make sure you're using these skills whenever needed.

☐ **Set new priorities.** If your stress is connected to an overly busy schedule or obligations that weigh too heavily on you, go back to My Priority Chart on page 57. Ask your diet coach for help in figuring out which activities you can eliminate, decrease, put off, or delegate.

☐ **Relax.** Take time to refresh yourself. Put "relaxation" in the essential column of your priority list and carve out at least one 20-minute period each day for some personal quiet time. Make sure to include this on your daily schedule until it becomes a habit. During this time, you can do yoga, take a hot bath, watch TV, read, meditate, listen to a CD or audiotape with relaxation exercises, write in a diary, or take a stroll and appreciate nature. Figure out an activity that clears your mind and relaxes you. I'd also like you to use relaxation techniques, such as slow, shallow breathing or stretching while you take slow, deep breaths—which you can do anytime, anywhere.

☐ **Get a good night's sleep.** Life is always more stressful when you're sleep deprived. (And a recent study showed that sleep deprivation alters hormones, increases appetite, and could contribute to being overweight.) Rearrange your schedule if you're not getting enough sleep.

☐ **Loosen rigid self-imposed rules.** Many chronically stressed people have unrealistically high standards for themselves and/or others, which leads to increased stress or anxiety when these rules inevitably are not followed. Loosening rigid rules is an important technique to increase personal satisfaction and to reduce overall stress. This is illustrated by the following three dieters and their expectations:

• *My rule is that my children must be high achievers at school.*

• *I have to be utterly perfect at work.*

• *I should do my absolute best at everything I do.*

Think about your expectations for yourself and others. What rules do you have that are stressing you out?

At home: _____

At work: _____

With your family: _____

With your friends: _____

With your community: _____

To change these rules, do the following:

☐ Consider people you know who have more relaxed standards than you. What are their rules?

_____

_____

☐ Think about whether you would want your best friend to be driven by these rules. What rules would you like him/her to have? _____

_____

_____

☐ Make a list of all the advantages you would reap by relaxing your rules: _____

_____

_____

☐ Add the word *reasonable* to your rules (*I should keep the house reasonably neat):* _____

_____

_____

what are you thinking?

Sabotaging Thought: If I relax my rules, things will fall apart.

Helpful Response: I'm not abandoning my rules, just making them more flexible. If problems arise, I can solve them when they do.

today's to-do list

Each night, remember to check off each task you've completed. Circle any you didn't do, so you can be aware that you didn't follow the program completely.

☐ I weighed myself.

☐ I read my list of reasons to lose weight (and other Response Cards as needed).

☐ I scheduled exercise and dieting activities on My Daily Schedule.

☐ I measured all of my food.

☐ I ate everything slowly and mindfully while sitting down.

☐ I refrained from overeating.

☐ I filled in my food plan *immediately* after eating.

☐ I said NO CHOICE to food that I wasn't supposed to eat.

☐ I stayed within my allotted units (calories, carbs, assigned points).

☐ I exercised (for at least 5 to 30 minutes).

☐ I used distraction techniques when I was hungry or having a craving.

☐ I contacted my diet coach if I needed help.

☐ I was alert for "fooling myself" thoughts.

☐ I used the *Oh, well* technique to deal with disappointment (if needed).

☐ I took steps to de-stress my life.

☐ I filled in My Daily Food Plan Chart (page 217) for tomorrow's meals.

☐ I gave myself credit for these things and for: _____

_____

_____

_____

_____

_____.

journal:

What did I do today to avoid unplanned eating? _____

_____

_____

_____

If I deviated, what happened? _____

_____

_____

_____

What sabotaging thoughts did I have? _____

_____

_____

_____

How did I answer back to them? _____

_____

_____

_____

What can I learn from this for next time? _____

_____

_____

_____

Reflections: _____

_____

_____

_____

_____

My Daily Schedule

Use this chart to plan your diet and exercise activities for today.

Time	Activity
6:00 a.m.	
6:30	
7:00	
7:30	
8:00	
8:30	
9:00	
9:30	
10:00	
10:30	
11:00	
11:30	
Noon	
12:30 p.m.	
1:00	
1:30	
2:00	
2:30	
3:00	
3:30	
4:00	
4:30	
5:00	
5:30	
6:00	
6:30	
7:00	
7:30	
8:00	
8:30	
9:00	
9:30	
10:00	
10:30	
11:00	

My Daily Food Plan Chart

units allowed: _____ calories/carbs/assigned points

| | | | Planned Eating | | | | Unplanned Eating | |
		Fill In Day Before and Check Off Immediately After Eating					Add Immediately After Eating	
	List Food	Amount	Units (calories, carbs, assigned points)	☑	List Food	Amount	Units (calories, carbs, assigned points)
breakfast							
snack							
lunch							
snack							
dinner							
snack							

units consumed: _____ calories/carbs/assigned points

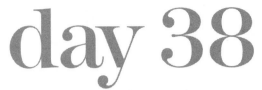

day 38

Manage Plateaus

If you have more than 15 to 20 pounds to lose, you may find that you reach a plateau after several months and don't lose any weight for several weeks. This is common and may be a sign that you no longer need as many calories as you have been taking in. If this happens, you have five options:

1. Continue doing exactly what you have been doing and see what happens.

2. Go back to carefully monitoring and weighing every bite of food to ensure you're sticking to the parameters of your diet plan.

3. Cut your intake by 100 to 200 calories per day, if your health-care professional approves.

4. Increase your daily exercise by 15 to 20 minutes.

5. Think of your present weight as your goal and move on to maintenance. (See "Transition from Losing to Maintaining" on pages 247–253 of this workbook.)

Finally, give yourself credit for everything you have accomplished to this point—and understand that a plateau is part of the process of losing weight. Don't let it discourage you; view it as an opportunity to review your diet, weight, and expectations.

what are you thinking?

Sabotaging Thought: I can't believe I hit a plateau, I knew this would happen. I'll never lose the rest of the excess weight.

Helpful Response: I will continue to lose if I eat less and/or exercise more. If it's not realistic or healthy for me to do that, I will need to work on being proud of the weight I've lost so far and to accept reality.

today's to-do list

Each night, remember to check off each task you've completed. Circle any you didn't do, so you can be aware that you didn't follow the program completely.

☐ I weighed myself.

☐ I read my list of reasons to lose weight (and other Response Cards as needed).

☐ I scheduled exercise and dieting activities on My Daily Schedule.

☐ I measured all of my food.

☐ I ate everything slowly and mindfully while sitting down.

☐ I refrained from overeating.

☐ I filled in my food plan *immediately* after eating.

☐ I said NO CHOICE to food that I wasn't supposed to eat.

☐ I stayed within my allotted units (calories, carbs, assigned points).

☐ I exercised (for at least 5 to 30 minutes).

☐ I used distraction techniques when I was hungry or having a craving.

☐ I contacted my diet coach if I needed help.

☐ I was alert for "fooling myself" thoughts.

☐ I used the *Oh, well* technique to deal with disappointment (if needed).

☐ I prepared myself mentally for a potential plateau in the future.

☐ I filled in My Daily Food Plan Chart (page 222) for tomorrow's meals.

☐ I gave myself credit for these things and for: _____

_____

_____

_____

_____.

journal:

What did I do today to avoid unplanned eating? _____

_____

_____

_____

If I deviated, what happened? _____

_____

_____

_____

What sabotaging thoughts did I have? _____

_____

_____

_____

How did I answer back to them? _____

_____

_____

_____

What can I learn from this for next time? _____

_____

_____

_____

Reflections: _____

_____

_____

_____

_____

My Daily Schedule

Use this chart to plan your diet and exercise activities for today.

Time	Activity
6:00 a.m.	
6:30	
7:00	
7:30	
8:00	
8:30	
9:00	
9:30	
10:00	
10:30	
11:00	
11:30	
Noon	
12:30 p.m.	
1:00	
1:30	
2:00	
2:30	
3:00	
3:30	
4:00	
4:30	
5:00	
5:30	
6:00	
6:30	
7:00	
7:30	
8:00	
8:30	
9:00	
9:30	
10:00	
10:30	
11:00	

My Daily Food Plan Chart

units allowed: _____ calories/carbs/assigned points

	Planned Eating — Fill In Day Before and Check Off Immediately After Eating				Unplanned Eating — Add Immediately After Eating		
	List Food	Amount	Units (calories, carbs, assigned points)	☑	List Food	Amount	Units (calories, carbs, assigned points)
breakfast							
snack							
lunch							
snack							
dinner							
snack							

units consumed: _____ calories/carbs/assigned points

day 39

Maintain Your Exercise Schedule

Maintaining a regular exercise regimen for a lifetime can be as difficult for some people as sticking to a diet. It takes time, energy, and persistence. Are you an all-or-nothing exerciser? Either you're 100 percent conscientious or you stop exercising altogether? Whenever you're tempted to stop, do the following:

☐ Remind yourself of all of the health benefits of exercise, not only now but also as you grow older.

☐ Read Response Card #7 ("Exercise No Matter What") twice a day.

☐ Go back to scheduling your life around exercise, as you did when you started out on Day 9 (page 59).

Here are some additional ideas to make it more likely that you'll exercise for the long term. Check off the ones that you need to work on:

☐ **Make exercise convenient.** Give yourself more than one exercise option. Always have a Plan B— and even a Plan C—for exercise. If you can't make it to an exercise class or to the gym, for example, take a walk or go for a bicycle ride outside. If the weather is bad, have a couple of DVDs and some hand weights and other inexpensive exercise equipment at home so you can get your exercise with them.

☐ **Always have your exercise clothing ready to go.** If you exercise in the morning, get your clothes ready the night before—if you see them, you're more likely to get yourself started. Pack up your bag with fresh clothes as soon as you get home from the gym. Keep an extra pair of running shoes in the trunk of your car.

☐ **Make sure you like your workout clothes.** Treat yourself to new exercise clothes, ones you really like and feel comfortable in.

☐ **Change your routine.** Change what you're doing from time to time so you can exercise other muscle groups and continue to get a good workout. Challenge yourself! If you do the same thing every day, your muscles adjust and stop working as hard.

☐ **Expand your definition of exercise.** You don't have to work out at a gym or to an aerobics tape. Movement comes in many forms, including dancing, playing tennis, jumping rope, and swimming. All of it counts! What do you like to do? A dieter I worked with found that it was easy and enjoyable to walk a lot—after she got a dog.

☐ **Exercise in a group.** The motivation and camaraderie that comes from exercising in a class or with a friend helps many people stick with their exercise program. After all, if you know you are going to see new friends or get together with an old one, you're more likely to show up. Socializing and being with others is a great motivator and can be part of the enjoyment of exercise. If you can afford it, hire a personal trainer. If you're paying for it, you'll feel more of an obligation to keep an appointment.

☐ **Put exercise firmly in your NO CHOICE category.** Rearrange your priorities and life demands, if necessary, but make sure that exercise is always at the top of the list of things that *must* get done.

what are you thinking?

Sabotaging Thought: I'm too busy to exercise.

Helpful Response: Why cut out exercise? Why not cut out or reduce other activities? Exercise is essential for my well-being. And it's not all or nothing. I have to remember that even five minutes is better then zero minutes when it comes to exercise.

today's to-do list

Each night, remember to check off each task you've completed. Circle any you didn't do, so you can be aware that you didn't follow the program completely.

☐ I weighed myself.

☐ I read my list of reasons to lose weight (and other Response Cards as needed).

☐ I scheduled exercise and dieting activities on My Daily Schedule.

☐ I measured all of my food.

☐ I ate everything slowly and mindfully while sitting down.

☐ I refrained from overeating.

☐ I filled in my food plan *immediately* after eating.

☐ I said NO CHOICE to food that I wasn't supposed to eat.

☐ I stayed within my allotted units (calories, carbs, assigned points).

☐ I exercised (for at least 5 to 30 minutes).

☐ I used distraction techniques when I was hungry or having a craving.

☐ I contacted my diet coach if I needed help.

☐ I was alert for "fooling myself" thoughts.

☐ I used the *Oh, well* technique to deal with disappointment (if needed).

☐ I got back on track with exercise.

☐ I filled in My Daily Food Plan Chart (page 228) for tomorrow's meals.

☐ I gave myself credit for these things and for: _____

_____

_____

_____

_____

_____ .

journal:

What did I do today to avoid unplanned eating? _____

_____

_____

_____

If I deviated, what happened? _____

_____

_____

_____

What sabotaging thoughts did I have?_____

_____

_____

_____

How did I answer back to them? _____

_____

_____

_____

What can I learn from this for next time? _____

_____

_____

_____

Reflections: _____

_____

_____

_____

_____

_____

My Daily Schedule

Use this chart to plan your diet and exercise activities for today.

Time	Activity
6:00 a.m.	
6:30	
7:00	
7:30	
8:00	
8:30	
9:00	
9:30	
10:00	
10:30	
11:00	
11:30	
Noon	
12:30 p.m.	
1:00	
1:30	
2:00	
2:30	
3:00	
3:30	
4:00	
4:30	
5:00	
5:30	
6:00	
6:30	
7:00	
7:30	
8:00	
8:30	
9:00	
9:30	
10:00	
10:30	
11:00	

My Daily Food Plan Chart

units allowed: _____ calories/carbs/assigned points

		Planned Eating Fill In Day Before and Check Off Immediately After Eating				**Unplanned Eating** Add Immediately After Eating		
		List Food	Amount	Units (calories, carbs, assigned points)	☑	List Food	Amount	Units (calories, carbs, assigned points)
breakfast								
snack								
lunch								
snack								
dinner								
snack								

units consumed: _____ calories/carbs/assigned points

day 40

Expand Your Horizons

Many dieters believe that they shouldn't pursue new interests and goals until *after* they have lost excess weight. But I don't want you to put your life on hold! I want you to really start living fully right away. Read Response Card #24 ("Enrich My Life Today"). To get you thinking, do the following:

☐ Look at My Enrichment Activities Chart on page 230 and then check off each item that represents an area where you could enrich your life.

☐ Write next to each checked item the specific steps you could take. For example, if you checked that you wanted to look for a new job, you might write, "I could start networking with people, go online to look for job openings, and post my résumé." If you checked that you wanted to join a group, club, or team, you might write, "I could check with my friends about a book group, with my church about social groups, and with the YMCA about a softball league."

☐ Add other things you'd like to do at the bottom of the list. If you're stuck for ideas, call your diet coach. Or discuss with other friends what *they* do.

Expanding your activities lifts your mood and gives you lots of non-food-related opportunities for pleasure and satisfaction. Improving your life actually increases your chances of diet success! And, besides, life is too short not to "seize the moment" and pursue your dreams and desires.

My Enrichment Activities Chart

Check off each item that could potentially improve your life and write down the specific steps you could take.

☐ Traveling _____

☐ Buying new, more fashionable clothes _____

☐ Taking up a hobby _____

☐ Signing up for a class _____

☐ Improving your work situation _____

☐ Looking for a new job _____

☐ Dating _____

☐ Joining a group, club, or team _____

☐ Going to the beach _____

☐ Making social plans with new people _____

☐ Volunteering _____

☐ _____

☐ _____

☐ _____

☐ _____

☐ _____

☐ _____

☐ _____

☐ _____

☐ _____

☐ _____

☐ _____

☐ _____

☐ _____

☐ _____

☐ _____

☐ _____

☐ _____

what are you thinking?

Sabotaging Thought: I'm still too heavy to enjoy life. I'll feel too self-conscious to try any of these new things.

Helpful Response: There shouldn't be any connection between how much someone weighs and what he/she does. Weight just isn't relevant. I shouldn't stigmatize myself for the way I look. I'm no different from anyone else, and I deserve to start having a better life—right now.

today's to-do list

Each night, remember to check off each task you've completed. Circle any you didn't do, so you can be aware that you didn't follow the program completely.

☐ I weighed myself.

☐ I read my list of reasons to lose weight (and other Response Cards as needed).

☐ I scheduled exercise and dieting activities on My Daily Schedule.

☐ I measured all of my food.

☐ I ate everything slowly and mindfully while sitting down.

☐ I refrained from overeating.

☐ I filled in my food plan *immediately* after eating.

☐ I said NO CHOICE to food that I wasn't supposed to eat.

☐ I stayed within my allotted units (calories, carbs, assigned points).

☐ I exercised (for at least 5 to 30 minutes).

☐ I used distraction techniques when I was hungry or having a craving.

☐ I contacted my diet coach if I needed help.

☐ I was alert for "fooling myself" thoughts.

☐ I used the *Oh, well* technique to deal with disappointment (if needed).

☐ I created a list of activities to enrich my life now.

☐ I filled in My Daily Food Plan Chart (page 235) for tomorrow's meals.

☐ I gave myself credit for these things and for: _____

_____

_____

_____

_____

_____.

journal:

What did I do today to avoid unplanned eating? _____

_____

_____

_____

If I deviated, what happened? _____

_____

_____

_____

What sabotaging thoughts did I have? _____

_____

_____

_____

How did I answer back to them? _____

_____

_____

_____

What can I learn from this for next time? _____

_____

_____

_____

Reflections: _____

_____

_____

_____

_____

My Daily Schedule

Use this chart to plan your diet and exercise activities for today.

Time	Activity
6:00 a.m.	
6:30	
7:00	
7:30	
8:00	
8:30	
9:00	
9:30	
10:00	
10:30	
11:00	
11:30	
Noon	
12:30 p.m.	
1:00	
1:30	
2:00	
2:30	
3:00	
3:30	
4:00	
4:30	
5:00	
5:30	
6:00	
6:30	
7:00	
7:30	
8:00	
8:30	
9:00	
9:30	
10:00	
10:30	
11:00	

My Daily Food Plan Chart

units allowed: _____ calories/carbs/assigned points

	Planned Eating Fill In Day Before and Check Off Immediately After Eating				**Unplanned Eating** Add Immediately After Eating		
	List Food	Amount	Units (calories, carbs, assigned points)	✓	List Food	Amount	Units (calories, carbs, assigned points)
breakfast							
snack							
lunch							
snack							
dinner							
snack							

units consumed: _____ calories/carbs/assigned points

day 41

Keep Your Skills Fresh

Spread the good news! If you teach what you've learned to someone else, you'll reinforce the important skills in your own mind. Think about who in your life might be receptive to learning the Beck Diet Solution: a friend, family member, coworker, or neighbor. Discuss the principles below:

- Dieting and exercise require significant time and energy.

- You need to eat a nutritious diet and modify it in advance to suit circumstances and preferences.

- You should arrange your home and work environments to reduce food triggers.

- It's better to waste food than to risk deviating from your plan.

- It's essential to learn the skills of writing down a food plan, monitoring food intake, and sticking to the plan—100 percent.

- Eating slowly and mindfully while sitting down needs to be a lifetime habit.

- Hunger and cravings are normal and tolerable. Certain activities can help you reduce these uncomfortable feelings.

- It's important to tolerate up to a 20-minute wait after eating for the sense of fullness to kick in.

- Weighing daily keeps you on track; expect normal weight fluctuations to avoid disappointment.

- You can learn to identify and counteract sabotaging thoughts.

- Life is sometimes unfair—so is dieting. You'll struggle less if you just say to yourself, *Oh, well.*

- It's important to give yourself credit for learning diet skills.

- When you make a mistake, face it and learn how to avoid mistakes in the future.

- It makes no sense to compound one mistake with another; get back on track immediately.

- Assertively say no to food pushers.

- It's important to seek out support and to ask for help when you need it.

- Plan for special events and traveling without blowing your diet.

- You can learn strategies to cope with negative emotions without turning to food.

- You can learn to handle disappointment and discouragement.

- You can learn to continuously motivate yourself to do all of these things.

today's to-do list

Each night, remember to check off each task you've completed. Circle any you didn't do, so you can be aware that you didn't follow the program completely.

☐ I weighed myself.

☐ I read my list of reasons to lose weight (and other Response Cards as needed).

☐ I scheduled exercise and dieting activities on My Daily Schedule.

☐ I measured all of my food.

☐ I ate everything slowly and mindfully while sitting down.

☐ I refrained from overeating.

☐ I filled in my food plan *immediately* after eating.

☐ I said NO CHOICE to food that I wasn't supposed to eat.

☐ I stayed within my allotted units (calories, carbs, assigned points).

☐ I exercised (for at least 5 to 30 minutes).

☐ I used distraction techniques when I was hungry or having a craving.

☐ I contacted my diet coach if I needed help.

☐ I was alert for "fooling myself" thoughts.

☐ I used the *Oh, well* technique to deal with disappointment (if needed).

☐ I taught what I've learned on the Beck Diet Solution to someone else.

☐ I filled in My Daily Food Plan Chart (page 240) for tomorrow's meals.

☐ I gave myself credit for these things and for: _____

_____

_____

_____

_____

_____.

journal:

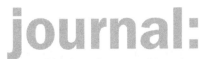

What did I do today to avoid unplanned eating? _____

_____

_____

_____

If I deviated, what happened? _____

_____

_____

_____

What sabotaging thoughts did I have?_____

_____

_____

_____

How did I answer back to them? _____

_____

_____

_____

What can I learn from this for next time? _____

_____

_____

_____

Reflections: _____

_____

_____

_____

_____

My Daily Schedule

Use this chart to plan your diet and exercise activities for today.

Time	Activity
6:00 a.m.	
6:30	
7:00	
7:30	
8:00	
8:30	
9:00	
9:30	
10:00	
10:30	
11:00	
11:30	
Noon	
12:30 p.m.	
1:00	
1:30	
2:00	
2:30	
3:00	
3:30	
4:00	
4:30	
5:00	
5:30	
6:00	
6:30	
7:00	
7:30	
8:00	
8:30	
9:00	
9:30	
10:00	
10:30	
11:00	

My Daily Food Plan Chart

units allowed: _____ calories/carbs/assigned points

	Planned Eating Fill In Day Before and Check Off Immediately After Eating				**Unplanned Eating** Add Immediately After Eating		
	List Food	Amount	Units (calories, carbs, assigned points)	☑	List Food	Amount	Units (calories, carbs, assigned points)
breakfast							
snack							
lunch							
snack							
dinner							
snack							

units consumed: _____ calories/carbs/assigned points

date: _____

day 42

Prepare for the Future

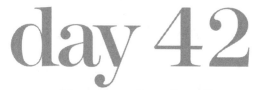

Congratulations! You have learned a set of powerful skills. In order to incorporate them fully into your life, you'll need to keep practicing these techniques over and over. Then you'll be ready for the tougher times. You'll know exactly what to do, and you'll get through these more difficult periods.

One of the most important skills you need to fortify is getting back on track. From time to time, you may eat things you hadn't planned or miss some exercise sessions. Forgive yourself when you make mistakes—but correct them immediately. Get out your Response Cards, reread sections of this workbook, and keep writing down what you can do to make positive changes. Like playing an instrument or a sport, dieting takes constant practice. Keep filling out your daily to-do lists, journals, schedules, food plans, and weight-loss graphs. (You'll need to make copies of each form; see pages 242–246.)

what are you thinking?

Sabotaging Thought: It's a lot of work to do these things forever.

Helpful Response: I don't need to use all of my skills forever, and the ones I do need will become more and more automatic. The results are worth it.

my daily to-do list

Each night, remember to check off each task you've completed. Circle any you didn't do, so you can be aware that you didn't follow the program completely.

☐ I weighed myself.

☐ I read my list of reasons to lose weight (and other Response Cards as needed).

☐ I scheduled exercise and dieting activities on My Daily Schedule.

☐ I measured all of my food.

☐ I ate everything slowly and mindfully while sitting down.

☐ I refrained from overeating.

☐ I filled in my food plan *immediately* after eating.

☐ I said NO CHOICE to food that I wasn't supposed to eat.

☐ I stayed within my allotted units (calories, carbs, assigned points).

☐ I exercised (for at least 5 to 30 minutes).

☐ I used distraction techniques when I was hungry or having a craving.

☐ I contacted my diet coach if I needed help.

☐ I was alert for "fooling myself" thoughts.

☐ I used the *Oh, well* technique to deal with disappointment (if needed).

☐ I filled in My Daily Food Plan Chart (page 245) for tomorrow's meals.

☐ I gave myself credit for these things and for: _____

_____

_____

_____

_____

_____.

my daily journal:

What did I do today to avoid unplanned eating? _____

_____

_____

_____

If I deviated, what happened? _____

_____

_____

_____

What sabotaging thoughts did I have? _____

_____

_____

_____

How did I answer back to them? _____

_____

_____

_____

What can I learn from this for next time? _____

_____

_____

_____

Reflections: _____

_____

_____

_____

_____

My Daily Schedule

Use this chart to plan your diet and exercise activities for today.

Time	Activity
6:00 a.m.	
6:30	
7:00	
7:30	
8:00	
8:30	
9:00	
9:30	
10:00	
10:30	
11:00	
11:30	
Noon	
12:30 p.m.	
1:00	
1:30	
2:00	
2:30	
3:00	
3:30	
4:00	
4:30	
5:00	
5:30	
6:00	
6:30	
7:00	
7:30	
8:00	
8:30	
9:00	
9:30	
10:00	
10:30	
11:00	

My Daily Food Plan Chart

units allowed: _____ calories/carbs/assigned points

	Planned Eating — Fill In Day Before and Check Off Immediately After Eating				Unplanned Eating — Add Immediately After Eating		
	List Food	Amount	Units (calories, carbs, assigned points)	✓	List Food	Amount	Units (calories, carbs, assigned points)
breakfast							
snack							
lunch							
snack							
dinner							
snack							

units consumed: _____ calories/carbs/assigned points

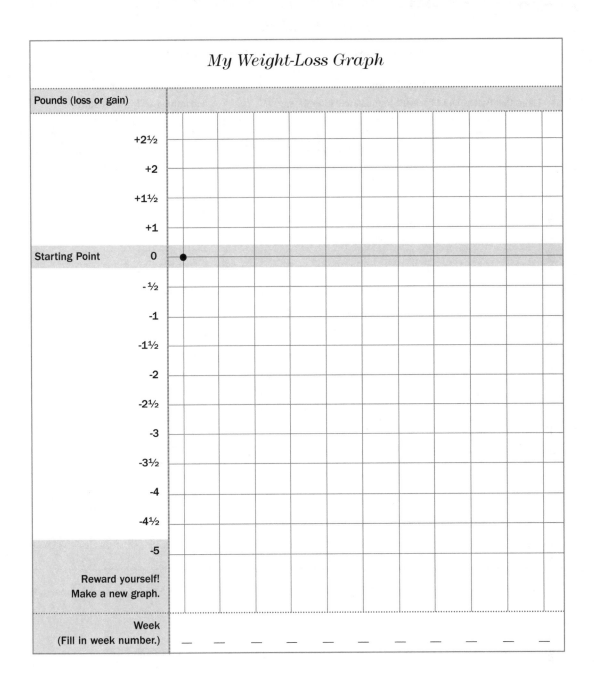

My Weight-Loss Graph

Pounds (loss or gain)											
+2½											
+2											
+1½											
+1											
Starting Point 0	●										
-½											
-1											
-1½											
-2											
-2½											
-3											
-3½											
-4											
-4½											
-5											
Reward yourself! Make a new graph.											
Week (Fill in week number.)	—	—	—	—	—	—	—	—	—	—	—

Transition from Losing to Maintaining

You've Changed!

This final section of the workbook will help you figure out how to go from dieting to rest-of-your-life eating. You'll find guidelines to assist you in determining the weight that you can maintain for the long term. And you'll learn what you need to do to make sure you're able to stay at that weight. Before you begin this section, though, I'd like you to go back and complete The Beck Diet Solution Questionnaire on pages 27–30 again, this time using a different color ink. If you've been faithfully doing the assignments in this program, I think you will find that you have made profound changes in your thinking and in your eating behavior.

Please take a moment now to journal about some of the changes you've made in your thinking and behavior:

journal:

_____

_____

_____

_____

_____

_____

_____

chapter 11

Transition to the Rest of Your Life

You've now been following the Beck Diet Solution program for six weeks—congratulations! Whether you're still losing excess weight or just working toward maintaining your weight loss, it's now time for you to learn how to develop a plan that you can follow for the long term—indeed, for the rest of your life! Now, do the following:

☐ **Wean yourself off any aspects of your diet that you don't think you can realistically keep up indefinitely.** For example, maybe you've been drinking a meal-replacement shake for breakfast or lunch. Start eating real food instead. If you've been depending heavily on prepackaged foods for lunch and dinner, start preparing homemade meals according to the calories and portions called for on your plan.

☐ **Develop a general plan for what you're going to eat every day.** For example, you may decide that you'll usually consume a predetermined number of calories for each meal and snack. You can experiment with not writing down this specific plan, not measuring out the foods, and not recording what you eat. Some people are able to transition to this kind of general planning at this point—but many cannot. So don't worry if you find you need to keep making a specific plan for a longer period of time.

☐ **Add to your list of reasons to lose weight.** Keep looking at your list periodically and record additional advantages. For example, see if any of the following apply: Are you less afraid of being hungry? Do you have fewer cravings? Are you more comfortable in social situations? Are you proud of yourself? Do you have greater enjoyment of the food you eat?

☐ **Keep weighing yourself every day.** Mark My Weight-Loss Graph (page 246) once a week and report your change in weight to your diet coach. Whenever your weight goes up by 3 pounds, go back to Day 1 (pages 39–40) and start practicing whatever skills are necessary to bring your weight back into check. Accept the fact that you'll need to be careful for the rest or your life. That's what anyone who has sustained significant weight loss has to do.

☐ **Give yourself lots of credit—again and again.** Never stop patting yourself on the back for all your hard work.

☐ **Continue to exercise.** You might want to change your routine from time to time to keep from getting bored and to make sure you work various muscle groups. How about taking up racquetball, water aerobics, or Pilates?

☐ **Ask for help.** Keep in touch with your diet coach for those times you need support.

chapter 12

Find and Maintain a Healthy Weight

S o how do you know when you've reached the point where you should transition to the maintenance phase of your diet? And how can you determine a realistic maintenance weight versus the (perhaps unrealistically low) number you have in your head? At some point in your dieting, you find that one of two things happens:

1. You reach a weight at which you are comfortable. If you haven't plateaued, you may be able to increase your calories modestly (perhaps by 200 to 400 calories per day) or to decrease your exercise and still stay at this weight.

   OR

2. You plateau but decide that even though you'd ideally like to lose more, you predict you won't be able to cut your calories any more or increase your exercise to levels you can sustain for the long term.

Determine Your Lowest Achievable Weight

If you have been at the same weight for two or more months, ask yourself the following questions:

- Do you want to reduce your calories even more?

- If so, could you sustain eating 100 to 200 fewer calories every day?

- Will cutting calories be healthy for you?

If the answer is no to any of these questions, it's time to change your focus. You have reached your "lowest achievable weight." Don't try to lose any more weight.

Determine Your Lowest Maintainable Weight

Once you've plateaued at your lowest achievable weight for several weeks, you have to make a decision. Can you easily keep eating and exercising the way you have been? If the answer is no, you should change your approach. Plan in advance to eat a little more (or exercise less) and accept that you will experience some weight gain—maybe 3 to 5 pounds or so. But I don't want you to just let your weight slide upwards by becoming looser with your eating or exercise. I want you to make a firm decision to change what you're doing and decide it's okay to gain a few pounds.

I Want to Be Even Thinner!

I often hear this lament from my unrealistic dieters. Even after you have reached your lowest maintainable weight, you might be thinking, *I would look better if I were thinner ... I'm not happy at this weight.* This is the moment to take stock: What does your health-care provider say about your weight? What do your friends and family think? Aren't others pleased and proud of you?

Rather than criticizing yourself, you need to work toward feeling satisfied with this weight you've worked so hard to achieve. If you're like 99 percent of humanity, you can't be model thin. You probably have a naturally bigger appetite, a slower metabolism, and a larger body frame than most models. You probably can't exercise as much as they do; you haven't had the cosmetic (body altering) surgery they've had; and you don't flirt with an eating disorder, as many of them do.

Don't let impossibly idealized images from the media make you feel bad about yourself. Instead, do the following:

☐ **Enrich your life.** Take time to take stock. Read Response Card #24 ("Enrich My Life Today"). Look again at the things you promised yourself you'd do only when you had lost weight and get started on doing them now: take a trip, build your career, have fun! Focusing outwardly gets you "out of yourself" and on to the things that make life important and pleasurable. Also decide how you can nourish yourself through relationships, volunteering and making someone else's life better, and connecting with your spiritual side.

☐ **Focus on your best features.** A lot of us, especially women, have a tendency to focus on the aspects of our bodies we like least. Instead, focus on the parts of your body you like *most*.

☐ **Say *Oh, well*.** Think about the other times when you have accepted the results of lesser goals in your life. Do you still struggle every day because you can't afford something you want or because your home isn't perfect? Or have you accepted the imperfections in your life? Why not say to yourself, *Oh, well, I've achieved a significant weight loss and this is how much I weigh ... I am not going to let it stop my enjoyment of life.*

☐ **Enjoy!** I hope you spend the rest of your life being proud of yourself for losing weight and keeping it off. It's really a magnificent achievement. Rejoice!

let's keep this going!

I would really love to hear from you. I learn so much from people who are actively dieting and maintaining. I'd like to know which parts of this workbook or *The Beck Diet Solution* were particularly helpful, as well as which perhaps were not. Tell me about your successes and challenges, tips that helped you lose and maintain your weight, and any other dieting ideas you have. Your input will allow me to help more dieters in the future. And as I learn more, I'll update our Web site: **www.beckdietsolution.com.** Visit it to contact me or write to me at:

The Beck Diet Program
P.O. Box 2673
Bala Cynwyd, PA 19004

Thanks! And I wish you all the luck in the world!
Judith Beck

Index

think

Response Cards

it's okay to disappoint people

I'm entitled to do what I have to do to lose weight, as long as I am nicely assertive.

say no to extra food

Get rid of extra food. It'll be wasted in the trash can or in my body. Either way, it's wasted.

put dieting first

I have to plan my life around exercise and dieting activities, not vice versa. I deserve to put myself first.

do it anyway

Even if I don't feel like using a diet skill, I have to do it anyway. If I do only what I feel like doing, I won't be able to lose weight and keep it off.

give myself credit

I deserve credit EVERY TIME I exercise. I deserve credit EVERY TIME I practice a dieting skill. I deserve credit EVERY TIME I stick to my plan.

eat mindfully

I need to eat slowly and mindfully while sitting down—EVERY SINGLE TIME.

if I'm hungry after a meal

Don't worry! It may take 20 minutes to feel full.

no excuses

Just because I want to eat, doesn't mean I should.

resistance habit

EVERY TIME I eat something I'm not supposed to, I strengthen my giving-in habit. EVERY TIME I don't give in, I strengthen my resistance habit.

exercise no matter what

If I don't feel like exercising, remember: 5 minutes is better than 0 minutes. Say NO CHOICE. The hardest part is getting started; then it gets easier.

tolerate it!

Hunger and cravings aren't emergencies. I can tolerate them. They're mild compared to _____.

I'm going to eat again in _____ hours, anyway.

distraction techniques

When I want to eat something I shouldn't, do these things instead:

_____

_____

_____

I'd rather be thinner

Being thinner is **SO** much more important

to me than eating this food.

NO CHOICE
NO CHOICE
NO CHOICE

get back on track

If I eat something I shouldn't have, I haven't blown it. It's not the end of the world. It's just a mistake. Get back on track this minute! Don't keep on eating! That makes no sense. It's a million times better to stop now than to allow myself to eat more.

can't have it both ways

I can be loose with my eating

OR

I can be thinner.

I can't be both.

it's not okay

It's **NOT OKAY** to eat this.

I'm going to be very sorry if I do.

I'll care later

I may not care right now, but I will care a **LOT** when I get on the scale.

be realistic

I shouldn't expect to lose weight every single week.

don't comfort myself with food

If I'm upset, don't eat to seek comfort! It won't solve the problem, and I'll just feel worse.

enrich my life today

I need to work toward developing a rich and rewarding life—right now.

celebrate!

I should celebrate each half-pound loss!

oh, well

I don't like this, but I'm going to accept it and move on.

advice to a friend

If my best friend were discouraged, disappointed, or dismayed, what would I tell him/her?